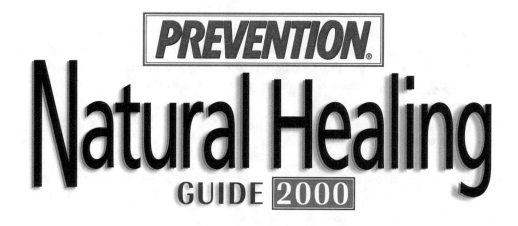

PREVENTION

Natural Healing

GUIDE 2000

Hundreds of Home
Remedies from America's
#1 Health Magazine

from the Editors of **Prevention** Magazine

RODALE

Notice

This book is intended as a reference volume only, not as a medical manual. The information given here is designed to help you make informed decisions about your health. It is not intended as a substitute for any treatment that may have been prescribed by your doctor. If you suspect that you have a medical problem, we urge you to seek competent medical help.

"The Art of Emotional Self-Defense" on page 206 is adapted from "It's the little things . . . that drive you crazy" by Ellen Michaud, which appeared in *Prevention* magazine, July 1998.

"The Healing Power of Prayer" on page 215 is adapted from "Do you have the miracle healer in you" by Ellen Michaud, which appeared in *Prevention* magazine, December 1998.

ISBN 1–57954–218–2 hardcover
ISBN 1–57954–256–5 paperback

Distributed to the book trade by St. Martin's Press

2 4 6 8 10 9 7 5 3 1 hardcover
2 4 6 8 10 9 7 5 3 1 paperback

Visit us on the Web at www.preventionbookshelf.com, or call us toll-free at (800) 848-4735.

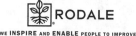

RODALE
WE **INSPIRE** AND **ENABLE** PEOPLE TO IMPROVE
THEIR LIVES AND THE WORLD AROUND THEM

Prevention Natural Healing Guide 2000 **Staff**

EDITOR: Doug Hill

EDITOR-IN-CHIEF, *PREVENTION* MAGAZINE: Anne Alexander

WRITERS: Anne Alexander; Alisa Bauman; Adam Bean; Susan G. Berg; Rick Chillot; Bridget Doherty; Varro E. Tyler, Ph.D., Sc.D.; Laura Goldstein; Sarí Harrar; Lois Guarino Hazel; Doug Hill; Jennifer L. Kaas; Mike McGrath; Eric Metcalf; Ellen Michaud; Arden Moore; Peggy Morgan; Deborah Pedron; Sara Altshul O'Donnell; Cathy Perlmutter; Shelly Reese; Judith Springer Riddle; Michele Stanten; Lee Tucker; Judith West; Selene Yeager

ART DIRECTOR: Darlene Schneck

INTERIOR DESIGNER: Richard Kershner

COVER DESIGNER: Christopher Rhoads

COVER PHOTOGRAPHER: Hilmar

PHOTO EDITOR: James A. Gallucci

ASSISTANT RESEARCH MANAGER: Shea Zukowski

LEAD RESEARCHER: Jennifer L. Kaas

SENIOR COPY EDITOR: Kathy D. Everleth

COPY EDITOR: Kathryn A. Cressman

EDITORIAL PRODUCTION MANAGER: Marilyn Hauptly

LAYOUT DESIGNER: Keith Biery

ASSOCIATE STUDIO MANAGER: Thomas P. Aczel

MANUFACTURING COORDINATORS: Brenda Miller, Jodi Schaffer, Patrick T. Smith

CONTENTS

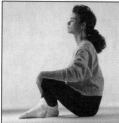

Ayurveda Explained:
What can India's science of life tell you about yourself?
PAGE 4

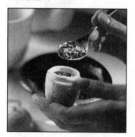

Natural Resource:
The government dishes out information on alternative medicine **PAGE 15**

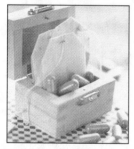

Herbal Knowledge:
How to tell a qualified herbalist from a quack
PAGE 21

iv

PART ONE

A Smart Guide to Alternative Medicine

A world of exciting new healing alternatives beckons. Here's how to find what you're looking for, safely.

PART TWO

Anti-Aging Secrets

The most long-lasting beauty comes naturally.
Stay young by applying some tender, gentle care.

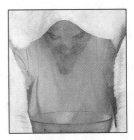

Steam Therapy:
Treat yourself to a
lavender, chamomile,
and rose facial
PAGE 30

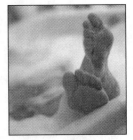

Foot Loose: Take
off the rough edges,
naturally **PAGE 34**

PART THREE

Healing with Vitamins

Vitamin and mineral supplements can build your body's
natural defenses against illness, boost energy, and
make you feel great.

**Put a Head
on It:** The
truth behind
the beer-
shampoo
stories
PAGE 41

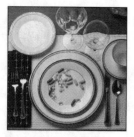

A Question of Timing: When is the right time to take your vitamins? **PAGE 49**

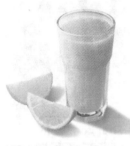

Vitamin C: More than just a cold remedy **PAGE 59**

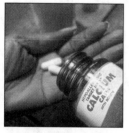

Supplement Safety: Here's what you need to know **PAGE 63**

PART FOUR

Miracle Foods

The same amazing powers that plants use to protect themselves can protect your health—and your family's.

PART FIVE
Modern Herbal Cures

For centuries, the healing powers of herbs have been mainstays of personal health. Now you can put that ancient wisdom to work in your home.

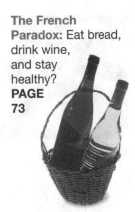

The French Paradox: Eat bread, drink wine, and stay healthy? **PAGE 73**

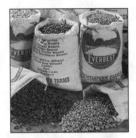

Small but Powerful: Beans deliver a disease-stopping punch **PAGE 79**

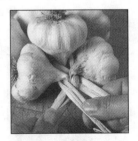

The Humble Healer: Roast garlic for health—and flavor **PAGE 87**

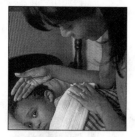

Rub It In: An aromatic herbal rub can soothe flu symptoms gently **PAGE 121**

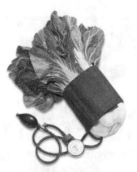

Heart Health: Some herbs are best not used to treat heart disease **PAGE 125**

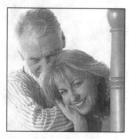

The Love Bug: An unexpected side effect from Viagra? **PAGE 137**

PART SIX
Natural Weight Loss

The natural route to getting slim is also the most effective route.

PART SEVEN

Fit and Firm— Naturally

In heaven, it won't be necessary to exercise.
Even in the real world, though, fitness can be
easy and fun.

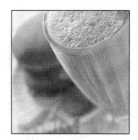

Why Do We Love Fat? Hint: It's more than just taste **PAGE 159**

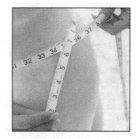

Yes, You Can: Stop playing the mental tapes that say "I can't" **PAGE 164**

Walk This Way: Perfect posture for the road **PAGE 180**

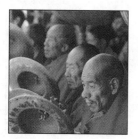

Mind over Matter:
Miracles from the
monks **PAGE 199**

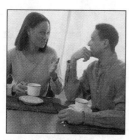

We Can Work It Out:
Surefire techniques
for peaceful commu-
nication **PAGE 207**

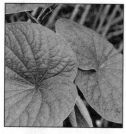

An Anxiety Herb:
Stressed to the max?
Kava can calm you
PAGE 212

PART EIGHT
Your Emotions and Your Health

The mind-body revolution shows that health
and happiness are intimately connected.

Chapter 20

You are what you eat—*and* what you think, what
you feel, and what you believe

Chapter 21

"Overeating nearly drove me to suicide, but I
fought my inner demons and won"

Chapter 22

Learning how to laugh at life's little irritations can
save your health

Hildegard of Bingen: A Healer Ahead of Her Time

Chapter 23

How fear works—and how you can chase it from
your life forever

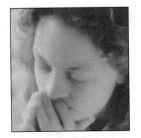

Faith in Healing:
Prayer is powerful
medicine **PAGE 215**

Introduction

Explore the Exciting New World of Natural Healing

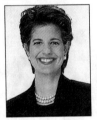

Welcome to the year 2000! The revolution in natural healing has been in full swing for at least a decade, and the impact that it has had on American health care is nothing short of astonishing. Now, at the turn of the century, is a terrific time to take stock of where we've been and where we're going. It's also a good time to put together, in one place, a compendium of the natural-healing knowledge that we've acquired so far—so that you can find exactly what you need, right when you need it. That's what this guide is all about.

I personally have been involved in the natural-healing movement for more than 10 years, and I still marvel at the diversity of health-care choices that have become available during that time. A quick turn to the Yellow Pages can put us in touch with herbalists who dispense remedies that were used by the pharaohs of ancient Egypt or pharmacists who sell vitamin supplements that first hit the market last week. Instantly, we can make appointments with acupuncturists or aromatherapists, herbalists or chiropractors, homeopaths or yoga instructors. And, of course, we can still talk with an old-fashioned M.D.

Our new ability to draw upon the whole history of human healing is a great privilege.

But it can also be confusing. The health-care marketplace of 2000 can be compared, for better and for worse, to a bustling bazaar where crowds of merchants shout for your attention—and your money. Their philosophies and techniques can complement one another, but they also compete. Informed choices need to be made.

Our goal with the *Prevention Natural Healing Guide 2000* is to give you an insider's advantage. Here you'll find thousands of practical tips and solutions, home remedies that work, dozens of herbal cures for your most common health problems, advice on how to buy and use herbs wisely, a complete rundown on finding the perfect vitamin supplements, a no-nonsense guide to losing weight naturally, the latest breakthroughs in natural nutrition, delicious recipes, and more. In short, the information packed between these two covers will provide you with a comprehensive, usable guide to the world of natural healing today.

Keep your *Prevention Natural Healing Guide 2000* right at your fingertips—and enjoy it in good health!

Anne Alexander
Editor-in-chief
Prevention magazine

An acupuncturist's needles can unblock the body's natural flow of life-giving energy, called *qi*.

Part One

A Smart Guide to
Alternative
Medicine

*A world of exciting new healing alternatives beckons. Here's
how to find what you're looking for, safely.*

Chapter 1

Navigating the Alternative Frontier

Who does what in alternative medicine, why they do it, and what to watch out for

At the dawn of the new millennium, a velvet revolution is overtaking American health care. Masses of Americans are seeking out and using alternative medicine. From herbal medicine to massage, from homeopathy to meditation, new and often exotic health-care modalities are increasingly welcome in our homes.

The problem is that, as a new frontier, alternative medicine is relatively uncharted territory. Those who have wanted to explore it have had to do so pretty much on their own.

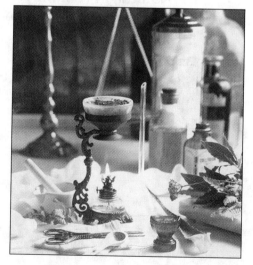

We'd like to help make subsequent navigation a bit easier. Here is a comprehensive road map of the different forms of alternative therapies that are out there, how they work, what they work for, and how to find people who practice them well.

Acupuncture: Ancient Wisdom That Heals

How can becoming a human pincushion possibly make you healthy?

The answer is that those hair-thin needles inserted just under your skin are actually stimulating the flow of a life-giving energy called qi (pronounced "chee"). In Chinese medicine, qi flows through invisible channels in your body, called meridians, to nourish your organs and limbs. These meridians can become blocked by unhealthy living or injury, which results in illness and pain. But when acupuncture needles are inserted at specific points along the meridians, say acupuncturists, the flow of qi is restored—as is your health.

As mystical as it sounds, this ancient treatment is actually well-researched and well-accepted. A consensus panel at our own National Institutes of Health (NIH) has concluded that acupuncture can help treat the nausea of pregnancy, chemotherapy, and surgery as well as postoperative dental pain. And although solid evidence is still lacking for other problems, some researchers feel that acupuncture may also relieve pain associated with arthritis, headaches, menstrual cramps, back pain, and fibromyalgia. It may even lessen the symptoms associated with withdrawal from drug and alcohol addictions.

Although many Western scientists still have trouble believing in qi, they know that acupuncture triggers the release of endorphins—your body's natural pain relievers. Plus, it may release a

The People's Choice

Why the surge in interest in alternative medicine? Here are some of the most commonly cited reasons.

We want alternatives. Conventional medicine does some things very well—treating heart attacks, fixing broken arms—but not everything. Alternative medicine shines where conventional medicine is weakest, especially in dealing with chronic ailments such as pain and depression.

We care about prevention. Conventional medicine focuses on fixing people who are sick. Alternative medicine pays more attention to keeping people healthy—and healthy means more than just feeling okay. The goal is optimal health: We want to thrive.

We want control. Many alternative practitioners encourage patients to participate in their own health-care decisions—a far cry from the condescending attitude of some conventional doctors.

We prefer natural remedies. Technology has worked wonders in medicine, but sometimes it seems to have taken over. The physical and psychological toll of surgical interventions and prescription drugs can be worse than the conditions they're meant to treat. Alternative treatments are usually gentler.

mood-lifting brain chemical known as serotonin and an anti-inflammatory known as cortisol.

As far as the actual needling is concerned, the needles themselves are extremely thin and flexible. So while they may sting a bit, they don't really hurt. Treatment lasts 15 to 60 minutes, and the acupuncturist may twirl the needles for greater effect. You should always insist that the practitioner use disposable needles to avoid infection.

The Basics

QUALIFICATIONS: Look for a practitioner with certification by the National Commission for the Certification of Acupuncture and Oriental Medicine (NCCAOM) or an M.D. with 200 hours of acupuncture training.

LICENSING: Most states provide licensing or certification.

NUMBER IN UNITED STATES: About 15,000 certified or licensed practitioners.

COST: $35 to $125 per session.

INSURANCE COVERAGE: Increasingly covered; check with your company.

FOR MORE INFORMATION: American Association of Oriental Medicine, 433 Front Street, Catasauqua, PA 18032.

Ayurveda: Be Yourself, Heal Yourself

Dubbed the science of life 5,000 years ago in India, ayurveda may be the oldest medical system in existence today. Its premise is that your body's

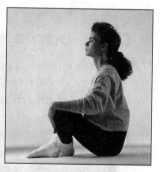

A Dosha Dictionary

Ayurveda is a lot easier to understand once you know which qualities in a person and which body functions are associated with each of the three ayurvedic categories. See which category you fall into.

Kapha: Water and earth; associated with the body's lubricating fluids. Caring, sensuous, centered, compassionate, good-humored, faithful, patient, down-to-earth, supportive. Kapha personalities tend to be steady and reliable, sometimes to a fault.

Pitta: Fire; involved with digestion, maintenance of body temperature, and assimilation of mental experiences. Ambition, passion, determination, confidence, enthusiasm for knowledge, happiness, intelligence. A pitta constitution tends to be alert and focused.

Vata: Air; involved with alertness and movement (circulation, reflexes, heartbeat, and so on). Creativity, enthusiasm, generosity, exuberance. Vata personalities are likely to be artistic and resourceful; actual execution of these ideas can be another matter.

biological intelligence (or ability to heal itself) acts through three forces called doshas. These are vata (space and air), pitta (fire and water), and kapha (water and earth).

All of us are made of a combination of these doshas, giving us a special metabolic type—or pakruti, as it's known in ayurveda. Most folks have one dosha that dominates and gives them characteristics associated with their primary elements. Vata people, for instance, are thin and energetic. Pittas tend to be hot-tempered. Kaphas are slow and solid.

So long as your doshas remain balanced, your health is fine, say ayurvedic doctors. But a diet of cheeseburgers, high stress, and even changing seasons can throw them off balance. And that's what causes the symptoms of disease. Generally, ayurvedic practitioners use herbs, meditation, exercise, diet, and other treatments to restore the balance of your doshas and make you well.

Ayurveda is best known for disease prevention, and 5,000 years of anecdotal evidence suggests that it can also treat many chronic diseases. Unfortunately, there are few medical studies to verify that, though some research has shown that meditation, exercise, and many of the herbs used in ayurveda will help lower blood pressure, cholesterol, and stress.

If you go to an ayurvedic practitioner, expect to spend 45 to 90 minutes answering all kinds of questions about your interests, emotions, and lifestyle. The practitioner will also take your pulse and may take urine, blood, or stool samples

NATURALFACT

Since 1990, use of herbal remedies in the United States has increased 380 percent, and use of vitamins for healing has risen 130 percent.

as part of the diagnosis. He or she may even ask you to stick out your tongue.

The Basics

QUALIFICATIONS: A bachelor of ayurvedic medicine and surgery (BAMS) degree from India, which equals 5½ years of medical school there. No schools in the United States offer that degree, though some offer courses on ayurveda as a specialty.

LICENSING: No licenses for ayurvedic practice are issued in the United States.

NUMBER OF PRACTITIONERS IN THE UNITED STATES: Unknown, but there are 10 clinics in North America.

COST: $40 to $100 for an initial consultation.

INSURANCE COVERAGE: Generally limited to M.D.'s or other licensed practitioners who specialize in ayurveda.

FOR MORE INFORMATION: The Ayurvedic Institute, 11311 Menaul Boulevard North East, Albuquerque, NM 87112.

Traditional Chinese Medicine: Staying in Balance

In the eyes of Traditional Chinese Medicine (TCM), every person is a miniature universe. You are yin and yang—two complementary forces like day and night. And your body is the interaction of five universal elements: water, fire, wood, metal, and earth.

All of these elements are pulled together by qi, that river of life-giving energy that flows through all of us. When it does its job and the elements are in balance, you have health, according to TCM. But when bacteria, an injury, or an unhealthy lifestyle throws them out of whack, you have disease—at which point a TCM practitioner's response will be to use acupuncture, medicinal herbs, massage, diet, and a movement meditation such as tai chi to restore balance and, consequently, health.

Since doctors can't find yin, yang, fire, or qi on an x-ray, TCM as a system is impossible to study by Western standards. What can be studied is the effectiveness of individual treatments like acupuncture and Chinese herbs. Acupuncture has been extensively researched and found to be useful for a variety of conditions. And, though more research is needed, various Chinese herbs may help alleviate a wide range of conditions, too.

One major caution surrounding TCM is to not use Chinese herbs, which you can buy in many Chinese markets, without first checking them out with a qualified practitioner. Many are potentially toxic and can be dangerous if you take them improperly.

If you make an appointment with a TCM practitioner, expect to answer questions about everything from your sleeping patterns to the color and consistency of your menstrual flow. The doctor will inspect your skin, hair, and tongue; listen to your voice and breathing; and check your pulse.

The Basics

QUALIFICATIONS: Look for certification by the National Commission for the Certification for Acupuncture and Oriental Medicine

Symbolic Meanings

We're all familiar with the yin-yang sign, a key symbol of the principle of balance that underlies Traditional Chinese Medicine. But do you know what the respective sides mean? Here are some of the qualities that yin and yang represent.

Yin	Yang
Moon	Sun
Rest	Activity
Earth	Heaven
Flat	Round
Space	Time
Cold	Hot
Inhibition	Excitement
Right	Left
Water	Fire

(NCCAOM) or a doctor of oriental medicine (D.O.M.) degree.

LICENSING: Licensing varies widely. Call the American Association of Oriental Medicine for the rules in your state.

NUMBER IN THE UNITED STATES: Unknown. Estimates are as high as 8,000.

COST: $75 to $150 for an initial visit; $25 to $100 for follow-up.

INSURANCE COVERAGE: Insurance coverage varies widely; check with your company.

FOR MORE INFORMATION: American Association of Oriental Medicine, 433 Front Street, Catasauqua, PA 18032.

Naturopathic Medicine: Enjoy an Eclectic Approach

Naturopaths are the symphony conductors of alternative medicine, capable of orchestrating a broad range of alternative therapies to prevent illness and treat it when it occurs. Acupuncture, herbs, diet, nutritional supplements, exercise, homeopathy, massage, and spinal manipulation may all be included in a naturopath's repertoire. All of these individual remedies have evidence to back them up, but because naturopathy incorporates such a vast array of therapies, there are no studies to show how effective it is as a whole.

Like other alternative practitioners, naturopathic physicians (naturopaths) pride themselves on harnessing your body's power to heal itself.

Drugs, therefore, are generally used as a last resort, although some states do give naturopaths limited prescribing authority.

If you decide to try a naturopath, you may have to search for a practitioner, since there are only about 1,500 in the United States. Once you've found one, however, expect to spend at least an hour at your initial visit, talking about all the factors that can affect your health, including exercise, diet, medical history, genetics, stress, exposure to pollutants, and emotional status. You'll also find many tests you'll recognize, such as x-rays, blood tests, and urinalysis. But when necessary, naturopathic physicians will refer you to M.D.'s and other health-care professionals.

The Basics

QUALIFICATIONS: Look for a licensed doctor of
naturopathy (N.D.).

HEALING SPOTLIGHT
Jane Seymour

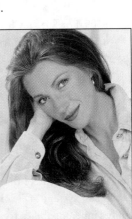

You know her as *Dr. Quinn, Medicine Woman*. What you may not know is that actress Jane Seymour is an alternative medicine woman in real life. Vitamins and herbal remedies play major roles in the health-care regimen of Seymour and her family, as does homeopathy. We asked her why she started using homeopathic remedies.

"I used to get a lot of colds and flu. Also, I'm allergic to some antibiotics. I break out in a red rash, which doesn't look good on TV. So I knew I couldn't rely on antibiotics every time I got sick. Even our pediatrician suggested we try homeopathic remedies with the babies because she felt they worked very well for viral infections. I also like the fact that I'm not taking endless drugs to disguise my symptoms—I'm taking care of the core problem."

LICENSING: Regulation varies widely from state to state. Call the American Association of Naturopathic Physicians to find out the rules in your state.

NUMBER IN THE UNITED STATES: About 1,500.

COST: $30 to $175 for initial consultation.

INSURANCE COVERAGE: Many companies will cover naturopathic services. Call yours to be sure.

FOR MORE INFORMATION: The American Association of Naturopathic Physicians (AANP), 601 Valley Street, Suite 105, Seattle, WA 98109. For $5, they'll send you a national directory.

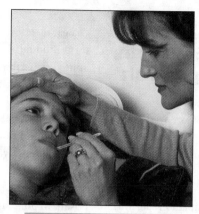

It is attention to detail that homeopaths say distinguishes their prescriptions from the "one diagnosis fits all" approach of conventional medicine.

Homeopathy: The Law of Similars

To its critics—and there are many—homeopathy is another name for snake oil. To its advocates—and there are many of those, too—it's a powerful yet gentle system of healing that stimulates the body's inherent ability to cure itself.

Homeopathy is based on the principle that like cures like (also known as the law of similars). Simply put, the idea is that certain substances create specific physical symptoms when taken by healthy people. If sick people who exhibit those same physical symptoms take small doses of the same substances, the thinking goes, their natural

defense mechanisms will be stimulated, and they will be cured. Homeopaths have more than 1,300 such substances, derived from plant, mineral, or animal sources, at their disposal.

In theory, it takes only minute amounts of these substances to trigger the body's healing response. Homeopathic remedies are prepared by diluting the active ingredient in water or alcohol, shaking it, and diluting it again. In many cases, these dilutions are repeated so often that no trace—not a single molecule—of the active ingredient remains. No matter: Homeopaths maintain that the remedies actually get stronger, not weaker, the more they are diluted. How exactly that occurs not even they can explain, although some research has shown that homeopathy is effective.

Homeopaths take great pride in pinpointing, exactly, each patient's specific problem. Like naturopaths, they see symptoms as signs of the body's natural healing process at work. Their goal is to help that process along, rather than to simply get rid of the symptoms. If you visit a homeopath for help with a chronic condition, expect to be grilled on everything from the color of the mucus you're spitting up to the times you break out in a sweat to the sorts of foods you crave. It is this attention to detail that homeopaths say distinguishes their prescriptions from the "one diagnosis fits all" approach of conventional medicine. There are also a number of standard homeopathic remedies for everyday ailments, which are sold in health food stores and national retail chains such as Kmart.

The Basics

QUALIFICATIONS: Several types of certification indicate a proficiency in homeopathy. Look for a physician who is a diplomate in homeotherapeutics (D.Ht.), a naturopath who is a diplomate of the Homeopathic Academy of Naturopathic Physicians (DHANP), or other practitioners who are certified in classic homeopathy.

LICENSING: Three states require licensing (Arizona, Connecticut, and Nevada). Other states allow providers to practice homeopathy as a specialty under another medical license, such as an M.D. or a D.O.

NUMBER IN THE UNITED STATES: About 3,000.

COST: About $140 for initial visit and $55 for follow-ups.

INSURANCE COVERAGE: Most insurance companies reimburse for homeopathy that is prescribed by a medical doctor or osteopathic physician. Call yours to find out.

FOR MORE INFORMATION: The National Center for Homeopathy, 801 North Fairfax Street, Suite 306, Alexandria, VA 22314. For $7, they'll send you an information packet that includes a list of practitioners.

‖ Aromatherapy: Soothe with Smell

The scent of roses, the smell of a pine forest, the aroma of an orange. All, according to aromatherapists, can be used to help heal.

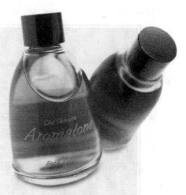

Smells Interesting

Scientists have had a hard time proving whether aromatherapy can actually cure illnesses, but there's little question that aromas do have some effect on our moods and our behaviors. Studies have found, for example, that:

• When specific aromas were pumped into a test site in a casino, gamblers spent up to 53 percent more money at the slot machines

• When a scent resembling the smell of baby powder was circulated in a hospital room, patients experienced less anxiety

• When fruity or floral scents were circulated in a jewelry store, people shopped longer. Pleasant scents also caused people to linger longer at museum exhibits

Aromatherapy uses pure essential oils distilled from plants and flowers. These oils are either diffused into the air so they can be inhaled, or applied to the skin by adding oils to the bath or through a massage with aromatic creams or lotions. Aromatherapists believe that each essential oil possesses unique healing qualities, and they recommend the oils for everything from arthritis and high blood pressure to fluid retention and cellulite, among numerous other health concerns.

Exactly how aromatherapy works—or whether it works at all—is hard to verify with traditional scientific methods. Still, plenty of research has documented the effect aroma can have on mood, which in turn may have a beneficial effect on health. "Anything that makes your environment more pleasant seems to be good for you emotionally," says Susan Knasko, Ph.D., an environmental psychologist at the Monell Chemical Senses Center in Philadelphia. "Therefore, aromatherapy has the potential to be an effective stress-buster. Scenting a room with a pleasing fragrance, taking a warm bath with a scent that you especially like, choosing music that relaxes you and lighting that soothes you—these are techniques that can help you gain control over a stressful environment."

The Basics

QUALIFICATIONS: Aromatherapists are certified by the American Society of Aromatherapy.

LICENSING: None.

NUMBER IN THE UNITED STATES: Approximately 5,000.

COST: $50 to $100 a session.

> ## NATURALFACT
>
> Acupuncturists are licensed in 32 states, naturopaths in 14, and homeopaths in 5.

INSURANCE: Aromatherapy is not usually covered by insurance.

FOR MORE INFORMATION: American Society of Aromatherapy, P.O. Box 95, Wallingford, PA 19086; or National Association for Holistic Aromatherapy, P.O. Box 17622, Boulder, CO 80308.

Osteopathy: A Structural Alignment

If you're basically comfortable with conventional care but wish your physician relied a little less on prescription drugs and a little more on hands-on healing, a doctor of osteopathic medicine or osteopathy (D.O.) may be the way to go. Osteopathic physicians (osteopaths) graduate from medical school, complete residencies, and pass certification exams just like M.D.'s. They can prescribe drugs and perform surgery. What D.O.'s have that M.D.'s don't have is specialized training in osteopathic manipulation—techniques for manipulating ligaments, muscles, and connective tissue, which osteopaths say can help the healing process.

Osteopaths believe that when it comes to health and healing, our musculoskeletal system gets short shrift. But by making sure all of your bones, vertebrae, ligaments, and tendons are lined up and working properly, say osteopaths, you can prevent and treat a host of conditions.

There's evidence that osteopathy may be effective for treating back, neck, and injury pain; headaches; and menstrual cramps. It may also help control other diseases like high blood pressure, arthritis, and digestive problems, though we need more research.

Unfortunately, research on osteopathy's effectiveness against any one specific ailment is in short supply. Osteopaths also admit that some people have more success with osteopathic manipulation than others, so you should be prepared to give it three to five treatments before you decide whether or not it works for you.

Since D.O.'s have the same training as M.D.'s, you can see an osteopath for any problem that you would call your family doctor for. If you go, expect your doctor to check the texture of your connective tissue, your posture, your range of motion, and other factors that reflect your skeletal health, and take your medical history. And he or she may prescribe anything from prescription drugs and manipulation to at-home exercise as your treatment.

Got It Covered?

If you're using alternative medicine, you may need to check out alternatives in health insurance as well. That's because most conventional health insurance policies still don't cover much more than traditional doctors, prescription drugs, and nonelective surgery, according to Michael Donio, director of projects for the People's Medical Society, a national health-care consumer-advocacy organization in Allentown, Pennsylvania.

One way to stretch conventional coverage so it includes alternative care is to find a traditional doctor who also uses those types of therapies. Most health insurance plans will cover trips to your M.D., whether she's the conventional type who prefers drugs or the holistic sort who recommends herbs, says Donio. Same goes for visits to doctors of osteopathy (D.O.'s).

Another way to maximize traditional coverage is to find an M.D. or D.O. with a practice that includes practitioners of herbal and other nontraditional treatments. A standard health policy should cover their services—if they're working under the supervision of the M.D. or D.O., says Robert McCaleb, president and founder of the Herb Research Foundation in Boulder, Colorado.

If you'd rather see a chiropractor, an herbalist, a naturopath, or a doctor of Oriental medicine as your primary-care physician, you may have to shop around for coverage. Some plans will cover some types of alternative medicine but not others. Even when alternatives are covered, there are often limits on the conditions or treatments for which you will be reimbursed.

For more information on how to get alternative medical bills covered, contact the People's Medical Society, 462 Walnut Street, Allentown, PA 18102.

The Basics

QUALIFICATIONS: Look for a doctor of osteopathic medicine (D.O.).

LICENSING: Osteopathic physicians are licensed in all 50 states.

NUMBER IN THE UNITED STATES: About 42,000.

COST: $55 to $95 per session.

INSURANCE COVERAGE: Reimbursement for osteopathic medicine is generally similar to reimbursement for conventional care.

FOR MORE INFORMATION: American Osteopathic Association, 142 East Ontario Street, Chicago, IL 60611.

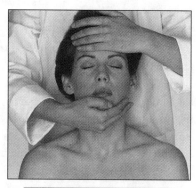

The chiropractor will push and pull on your joints and spine to correct your alignment.

common back pain is. It strikes about 80 percent of us at some point in our lives, which may explain why one in three of us has tried chiropractic care. The Agency for Health Care Policy and Research in Rockville, Maryland, has found that spinal manipulation is indeed a help for lower-back pain. However, there are no well-controlled studies to support manipulation for gastrointestinal, breathing, and other nonmechanical problems.

If you go, expect a very physical experience. The chiropractor will push and pull on your joints and spine to correct your alignment. You should give it 5 to 10 treatments before you expect to see results.

Chiropractic: Healing Adjustments

If there is strength in numbers, chiropractors are one of the strongest alternative medicine groups going. With more than 45,000 practitioners in the United States, they are second only to physicians in providing primary care. Though some chiropractors have been criticized in the past for trying to treat everything through spinal adjustments, today's chiropractors generally use adjustments to treat mechanical problems that you expect to respond to mechanical manipulation—headaches, neck pain, back pain, and pain from musculoskeletal injuries.

We probably don't have to tell you how

The Basics

QUALIFICATIONS: Look for a doctor of chiropractic (D.C.) who has passed the National Board of Chiropractic Examiners board exam.

LICENSING: Chiropractors are licensed in every state.

NUMBER IN THE UNITED STATES: Between 45,000 and 50,000.

COST: $50 to $100 for an initial visit and $25 to $65 for follow-ups.

INSURANCE COVERAGE: Most insurance, including Medicare and many state Medicaid programs, cover chiropractic.

FOR MORE INFORMATION: American Chiropractic Association, 1701 Clarendon Boulevard, Arlington, VA 22209.

NATURAL HEALING THROUGH HISTORY

Isis: The Divine Physician

Who founded the art of healing, and when?

If you answered Hippocrates, you were off by a couple of thousand years, at least. Hippocrates studied the medicine of the Egyptians, and the Egyptians credited the invention of medicine to Isis, divine physician and source of all healing herbs.

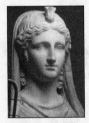 Isis was the most important and most revered goddess of all Egyptian mythology. She may have been born a mortal before being granted divinity as a reward for some great service. So great were her healing powers, and so long-lasting her influence, that even in the later days of the Roman empire, centuries after Isis emerged in Egypt, many preferred to continue worshipping her rather than the controversial new deity of that era, Jesus Christ.

Temples dedicated to Isis worship existed as early as 2,000 B.C. and were said to be magnificent, part religious shrine and part health spa. Ailing Egyptians traveled great distances in hopes of being healed by the temple priestesses, who kept secret lists of diseases and cures. Each of them specialized in treating a particular area of the body, just like our modern-day physicians. They were said to have been strict vegetarians with shaven heads, dressed in white linen and consecrated to purity.

Those seeking Isis's healing powers would bring offerings of food and clothing to her temple, where a wax model of the patient would be placed on the altar. Herbal medicines, massages, fasts, and healing baths would follow, augmented by complicated ritual performances of prayers, holy songs, and incantations. The priestess-healers were responsible for cultivating the temples' extensive gardens of medicinal herbs and for overseeing the preparation of remedies. Egyptian pharmacists used a broad assortment of mortars, mills, sieves, and balances to prepare more than 800 standardized prescriptions. Some historians believe that the modern-day Rx pharmacy symbol is derived from an Egyptian hieroglyph called the Eye of Horus.

Some of Isis's temples later became important medical schools, one of which was responsible for composing one of the oldest comprehensive medical texts that we have today, the Papyrus Ebers. Dated around 1550 B.C., the papyrus was dedicated to Isis. The following invocation to the goddess is found at its beginning.

"O Isis, thou great enchantress, heal me, deliver me from all evil, bad typhonic things, from demoniacal and deadly diseases and pollutions of all sorts that rush upon me."

Chapter 2

Dr. Natural, I Presume?

How do you find the right natural healer? We're glad you asked

Your Aunt Hilda says that one of her best friends just got a certificate in homeopathy. Should you trust auntie's friend? You meet an ayurveda practitioner who says that he was trained at something called the Acme Ayurveda Academy in Toledo, Ohio. How do you know if that's one of the best schools in the country or one of the worst?

The honest answer to these sorts of questions is that, many times, there are no definitive answers. The education required to become a certified practitioner of various types of alternative medicine varies tremendously. So do the licensing requirements in different states—if there are any licensing requirements.

Knowing where to look and what to ask can make finding the right alternative healer a lot easier, and a lot safer.

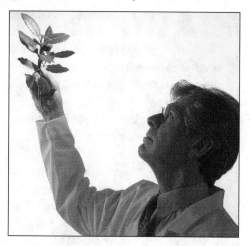

Where to Start

At this point in the evolution of the alternative movement, it's probably not a good idea to rely exclusively on alternative care for treatment of medical conditions, at least not until you've been checked out by a conventional M.D. That's why the trend is toward "complementary" or "integrated" medicine, which combines the strengths of both conventional and alternative medicines.

Starting your treatment with an M.D. who's receptive to alternative methods is a great choice. "Then you know that you're not going to miss something bigger," says Kathleen Fry, M.D., a homeopathic practitioner and gynecologist in Scottsdale, Arizona, and president of the American Holistic Medical Association. Patients with life-threatening illnesses should be referred to a conventional physician, Dr. Fry believes.

Ideally, your family doctor will be familiar with alternative practitioners in your area and can refer you to them as needed. If your medical doctor isn't quite there yet, you may have to build up the alternative side on your own. Here's how.

Call the authorities. To find out which types of therapists are licensed in your state, call the state board of medical examiners, your local or state health department, or your local representative in the state legislature, suggests Dr. Fry.

Ask a local merchant. People who work in quality health food stores are often knowledgeable about holistic healing practitioners in their areas, says James S. Gordon, M.D., director of the Center for Mind/Body

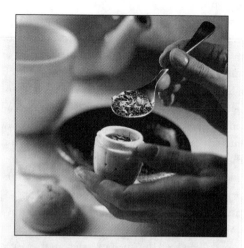

Natural Resource

A government source of general information is the Office of Alternative Medicine (OAM), which is part of the National Institutes of Health. The OAM doesn't make actual referrals, but it does publish a "General Information Package" that includes good advice on locating and selecting an alternative-care practitioner. Write to the OAM Clearinghouse, P.O. Box 8218, Silver Spring, MD 20907.

Medicine in Washington, D.C., and author of *Manifesto for a New Medicine*. In the days when he used to suffer from back pain, he made it a habit when traveling to ask at health food stores for leads on good chiropractors, osteopaths, or massage therapists. "I always found someone," he says.

Get online. Another invaluable source of information is the Internet. Some of the major national organizations have their own

Web sites, where you'll usually find plenty of material explaining what the therapy consists of and, often, referral information. Because Web addresses change so often, we can't list them here, but a browser search using the organization's name should get you there quickly enough. (See "Safe Surfing" for more on using the Internet wisely.)

Ask a friend. Word of mouth is a surprisingly reliable way to find an alternative practitioner you'll like, according to Dr. Gordon. "Yes, it's possible to get a bum steer from a friend," he says. "But the best referrals that I get in my practice come from other patients. They know who's going to work well with me because they know the kinds of things I ask patients to do and whether their friends will be ready to do them."

Grill 'em. Remember that when you agree to be treated by any health-care professional, you're hiring him or her. And like any prospective employer, you have a right to conduct a job interview. Asking some preliminary questions over the phone can rule out the obvious rejects, but when you're getting closer to making a decision, there's really no substitute for a face-to-face visit. Doctors call that a consultation, and it's reasonable to expect to pay for it. Rates will vary, but a fee of up to $100 for an alternative practitioner would be typical, estimates Wendy Wetzel, R.N., a family nurse practitioner, certified holistic nurse, and a longtime officer with the American Holistic Nurses Association. "It's well-worth the expense of a consultation to see if it's somebody you can work with," she says. "If someone doesn't want to do a consultation, look elsewhere."

Know what you want. Think about the kind of care you need and the type of

Safe Surfing

The Internet puts reams of material about virtually every health subject you can think of—from acupuncture to yeast infections—just a mouse click away.

How can a person become a savvy consumer of health information on the Internet? We put that question to the leading expert on Internet health, Tom Ferguson, M.D., editor and publisher of the *Ferguson Report* newsletter.

Dr. Ferguson believes that online discussion groups dedicated to specific health concerns are a rich new source of health-care information. He warns, however, that you need to approach these groups with caution and patience. "You have to spend some time on the Web," he says. "It's kind of a different world and you have to learn how it works. You can't uncritically accept everything that you see."

people you work best with before that first visit, suggests Adriane Fugh-Berman, M.D., chair of the National Women's Health Network and author of the book *Alternative Medicine That Works.* "Specifically, do you want someone who will be your health-care partner; or do you prefer a health-care professional who just tells you what to do? Not everyone who seeks out alternative care wants to make choices on his or her own

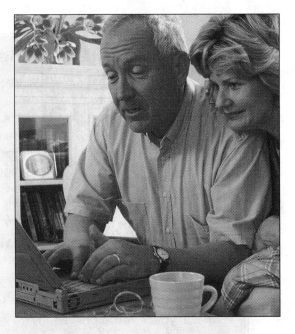

How do you know when you're getting good advice?

"There are a lot of quality-control resources on the Internet itself that you can use to check questionable information. For instance, in a lot of the discussion groups, any off-the-wall postings are pretty quickly jumped on. It's generally a good idea, if you're dealing with a chronic health concern, to find a community of people who share that concern. Just observe and listen in for awhile to get a feel for how the group works. When you feel comfortable, jump in and start participating."

What are some types of sources on the Internet that offer good, reputable advice?

"There are several characteristics of good advice. One is whether it's really patient-centered. A lot of information that may be technically accurate is really not presented in a way that is the most useful to the consumer. A lot of online self-helpers tell me they find materials developed by online self-help groups particularly useful because they are so targeted to patients' real concerns. A good tip if you're looking for a given concern is to do a search-engine search on your topic plus "support group" or your topic plus "self-help." Or search for your topic plus FAQ, for 'frequently asked questions.'"

or even be a part of the process—some people feel that being offered choices means that the practitioner doesn't know what to do." There's no right or wrong way—do what works for you.

Listen to your gut. Gathering information is important, but there's a limit to how far the just-the-facts-ma'am approach can take you. In the end, you have to rely on your instincts.

"You really have to use your intelligence and your intuition in deciding whether you want to go with any practitioner, alternative or conventional," says Dr. Gordon. "When you're asking your questions, listen to the content of the answers, but try to get a sense of what kind of person this is as well."

Keep everyone informed. If you're under a doctor's care for any medical

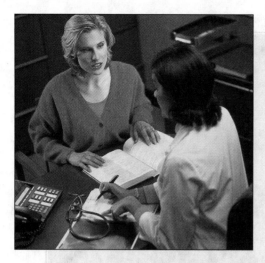

Be Prepared

When you interview an alternative practitioner, James S. Gordon, M.D., director of the Center for Mind/Body Medicine in Washington, D.C., and author of *Manifesto for a New Medicine*, suggests that you ask the following questions.

• Where were you trained?

• What degrees or certificates have you earned?

• How long have you been practicing?

• What professional associations are you a member of?

• What is your healing philosophy?

• Have you been able to help people with my condition in the past? May I contact some of them?

• Is there any research that shows that this treatment works for my condition?

• How long will it take before I see results?

• Are there any potential side effects or interaction with medicine that I'm already taking or treatment that I'm already getting?

• How much will each session—and any medication/supplements/herbs—cost?

condition, it's important that the lines of communication be open between your M.D. and any alternative therapist you go to. That's especially true if you're on medication and you're thinking of embarking on any course of herbal or nutritional therapy, says Dr. Fry. A few prescription drugs can interact dangerously with such treatments. Patients undergoing chemotherapy or radiation therapy, in particular, should exercise caution.

Chapter 3

Become an Educated Herb Consumer

Cut through the confusion to find the herbal remedy that's right for you

I t's a jungle in there.

Anyone who has ever taken a walk through the herbal-remedies aisles of the local health food store or drugstore knows that. A seemingly endless variety of concoctions clutters the shelves, each shouting a litany of claims and promises.

Determined to find some way to sort through the chaos, we asked one of the world's top herb experts, Varro E. Tyler, Ph.D., Sc.D., distinguished professor emeritus of pharmacognosy and dean emeritus of Purdue University School of Pharmacy and Pharmacal Sciences in West Lafayette, Indiana, and author of *The Honest Herbal*, for his advice in choosing where and how to buy herbal remedies. Here are his rules for shopping for herbs wisely.

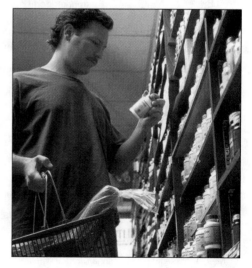

The Four Rules of Smart Herb Buying

Rule #1: Choose the herb that's right for you. First, ask yourself why you're buying a particular herb. Then make sure it's appropriate for the condition you're treating. Science has established the value and safety of numerous herbs for treating many common problems, such as black cohosh for menopausal symptoms, chasteberry for menstrual problems, licorice for coughs, and valerian to relieve insomnia. (See "Some Standardized Herbs at a Glance" for a list of other proven herbal healers.)

Rule #2: Look for standardized extracts. Herb quality varies widely depending on where it was grown, the time of harvest, the method of drying, and the length of storage. Even genetic composition comes into play. So it's obvious that ground or powdered herbs are also going to range considerably in their potency and efficacy.

A standardized extract is prepared so that a given weight of the product contains a specific amount of one or more of the herb's active constituents—the ingredients that give it its healing power. Alternatively, the product may be standardized for a so-called marker compound that is

Some Standardized Herbs at a Glance

Herb	Basis of Standardization	Helps Treat or Prevent
ECHINACEA	echinacosides (marker compound)	colds and flu
FEVERFEW	parthenolides (marker compound)	migraine
GARLIC	allicin yield	cholesterol, infections
GINKGO	flavonoids and ginkgolides	cognitive deficiency
GINSENG	ginsenosides	reduced vitality
GRAPESEED, GREEN TEA, OR PINE BARK EXTRACT	proanthocyanidins (many names)	oxidative tissue damage
KAVA KAVA	kavapyrones (kavalactones)	anxiety
MILK THISTLE	silymarin complex	liver disorders
ST. JOHN'S WORT	hypericin (marker compound)	depression
SAW PALMETTO	lipids and steroids	benign prostatic hyperplasia (prostate disease)

Many of these herbs are standardized at different levels of active or marker constituents. Therefore, it is difficult to recommend a standard dosage for each. The best advice is to take the amount recommended on the label.

believed to reflect the concentration of its active ingredients.

For example, one brand of ginseng is prepared so that each capsule contains 100 milligrams (mg) of herbal extract standardized to a level of 4 percent (4 mg) total ginsenosides—the main active constituent. Most standardized St. John's wort products are adjusted to contain a level of 0.3 percent hypericin. In this case, hypericin is a marker compound and not the

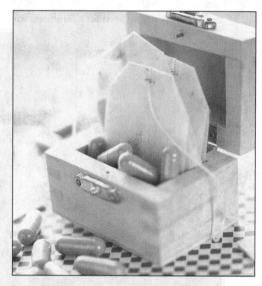

Hunting for Herbalists

How do you find a qualified herbalist?

Many naturopaths and doctors of Oriental medicine use herbs regularly in their practices and are likely to have developed significant expertise in the art of herbal medicine. Some chiropractors and some physicians—both M.D.'s and D.O.'s—have taken the time to learn about phytomedicines. In addition, you may find some pharmacists who are quite knowledgeable.

The gold standard in herbalism, however, is membership in the American Herbalists Guild (AHG). Not even a decade old, the Guild is 1,000 herbalists strong, and its members are "the only peer-reviewed organization of clinical herbalists" in the United States, according to David Winston, a co-founder of the AHG and founder of Herbalist and Alchemist, an herbal-medicine company in Washington, New Jersey. That means the members have to be judged to be competent practitioners by a panel of five AHG members.

Winston stresses that not every good herbalist out there is a member of the Guild. That's especially true because herbalism is populated by many unconventional types who aren't interested in joining organizations. If an herbalist you're considering doesn't have the AHG initials after her name, be prepared to make your own appraisal. And don't be afraid to ask for the names of others the herbalist has treated.

The AHG will provide you with a directory of all their members for $5; to obtain one, send a check to the AHG at P.O. Box 70, Roosevelt, Utah 84066.

principal active ingredient, which is still un-known.

Rule #3: Find the form that's right for you. People who have difficulty swallowing capsules or tablets may prefer a tincture of the herb, which is usually prepared with water and alcohol, or an extract. Tinctures or liquid extracts that use alcohol or other solvents to extract the herb's healing power are easy to take. The solvent (called a menstruum) dissolves the medicinal components so they can be easily absorbed by the body. Buy the freshest liquid product available; a good herbal tincture will have an expiration date.

Soothing herbal teas have been used as medicine for thousands of years. As long as an

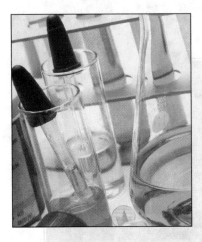

Calling Commission E

The United States is a groundbreaker in many fields, but not in herbal medicine. Many European countries are far ahead of us in using herbs, perhaps none more so than Germany.

In 1978, the German government established the somewhat sinister sounding Commission E to evaluate the effectiveness of herbal remedies. The commission, made up of physicians, toxicologists, pharmacologists, and other specialists, examined hundreds of herbs with an eye toward determining which ones worked, what they worked for, how best to use them, and how not to use them.

The commission's report—a thick tome of more than 680 pages—covers some 400 herbs. Its scientific standards are somewhat looser than the United States government would require: a finding of "reasonable certainty," rather than "absolute certainty," is deemed acceptable for judging an herb effective, for example. Traditional use and anecdotal evidence were also taken into account, along with scientific studies.

The results: Germans today have access to nearly 700 plant-based remedies; some 70 percent of German physicians routinely prescribe herbal medicines; and pharmacists there are knowledgeable about them as well.

herb's active constituents are water-soluble (able to dissolve in water), you can brew it into a tea. In general, herbs that are pleasantly aromatic make excellent teas. A very short list of good tea herbs includes ginger, fennel, chamomile, and various mints. Use approximately 1 teaspoon of dried herb to 1 cup of boiling water; steep, covered, for up to 15 minutes.

Some herbs, such as saw palmetto and milk thistle, have constituents that aren't water-soluble, so they won't do you any good as teas. Ginkgo shouldn't be made into a tea for two reasons: First, the unprocessed leaf contains toxic compounds related to those in poison ivy; theoretically, it could cause a reaction. Second, the tests done on ginkgo used a leaf extract concentrated to at least 50:1, so it's best to use products at that concentration.

Rule #4: Choose the best herb brands. The industry hasn't yet come up with a uniform way to test individual products. There are a variety of different testing methods, and they may yield different results. However, there's enough data to show that the quality of herbal products varies greatly. Admittedly, choosing a good brand can be difficult, but here are four additional rules that will assist even the most perplexed shopper.

1. Look for well-tested products. Many brands are identical to the form of herb that's proven itself in scientific testing. Usually, when a brand has been tested, you'll know it by reading the label. Examples include Ginsana ginseng, Kwai garlic, Ginkgold ginkgo, LeucoSelect grapeseed extract, Thisilyn milk thistle,

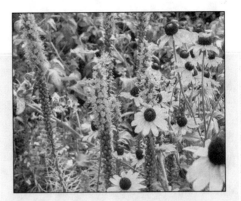

Naturally Complex

Nature has "programmed" plants with a miraculous array of chemical properties that combine to make up their healing powers. Each herb has a unique chemical fingerprint that may include hundreds or perhaps thousands of different substances. "We know now that a well-researched herb like licorice contains more than 600 different compounds, and there are still more to discover," says James Duke, Ph.D., a former ethnobotanist with the U.S. Department of Agriculture and author of *The Green Pharmacy.* "I think we will one day know that each herb actually contains thousands."

and Kira St. John's wort. This is just a small sampling. Other products may be equally good, but these are the ones that have solid research backing.

2. Choose a brand that's well-made. Herbal-product manufacturers are required to adhere to standards established for food processing (so-called food GMPs, or Good Manufacturing Practices). Some voluntarily adhere to higher manufacturing standards established for drugs (drug GMPs). Those that do are proud of it and may mention it in their catalogs or advertising.

3. Buy single-herb products that clearly indicate how much of the herb you get in a single dose. Complex mixtures containing numerous herbs often contain inadequate doses of each. As in most things, you generally get what you pay for; cheap herbs are not necessarily a good buy.

4. Finally, beware of outrageous claims. If an herb sounds too good to be true, it probably is. Don't buy products with "secret formulas," and think twice about products that aren't sold in health food stores or in other conventional retail outlets.

NATURAL HEALING IN THE FUTURE

Onward the Revolution

Equal parts crusader and guru, Andrew Weil, M.D., is arguably the single most prominent leader in natural healing today. Here the author of the bestselling books *Spontaneous Healing* and *Eight Weeks to Optimum Health* discusses his vision of the health-care future with *Prevention* editor-in-chief Anne Alexander.

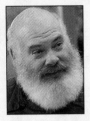

Q: How do you define "optimum health"?

A: In my view, health is a state of balance. It is the balance between the body's healing system and whatever outside stresses we come across. On a day-to-day basis, optimum health is that inner resilience that allows you to come into contact with millions of germs every day and not get an infection or to be exposed to carcinogens and not get cancer. It is what enables you to recover from illnesses or injuries or to handle ordinary stresses without throwing your digestion or blood pressure out of whack. Over time, it means not getting heart disease or cancer in middle age or being crippled by diseases like arthritis in later life.

But optimum health is also much more than just the absence of disease, it's a sense of strength and joy. However, it's not magic, either. Optimum health doesn't mean that you'll achieve immortality or find eternal happiness. Most likely, you won't even be aware of it, because we tend to ignore our health when it is good.

Q: Is the idea that the body has its own "healing system" your own theory?

A: No. It's as old as Hippocrates. Today, he is known for only one of his admonitions to doctors ("First, do no harm"), but he also had another very important piece of advice: "Honor the healing power of nature." Healing is a natural power that, unfortunately, is completely overlooked by conventional Western medicine. That seems to be the single greatest defect of modern medicine: We don't encourage the body's own healing potential.

Q: How may that be changing as we enter the new millennium?

A: In the future, I hope that there is a lot more research on alternative medicine. That's one of the reasons I started the program in integrative medicine at the University of Arizona College of Medicine in Tucson. This program is designed to train physicians to integrate the best of conventional and alternative medicine. In addition, the doctors in the program will be conducting research on the efficacy of different alternative medicine modalities.

The time is right for change and, I believe, the direction we need to move in is clear.

Beautiful skin
can be nurtured
from the inside
as well as from
without.

Part Two

Anti-Aging
Secrets

The most long-lasting beauty comes naturally.
Stay young by applying some tender, gentle care.

Chapter 4

The Natural Route to Radiant Skin

You don't need chemicals or surgery to have skin that glows with health

Age deserves respect. Wrinkles are meaningful signs of a lifetime's worth of lessons learned, of wisdom earned. So how come nobody wants them?

The great American obsession with youth may be lessening these days. Many of us are becoming more comfortable with the fact that getting older doesn't necessarily mean we have to sit around senior citizens' homes, reminiscing and watching TV. Scientists talk of the difference between "actual" age and "functional" age. It's entirely possible to feel 35 when you're actually 50. Seen in that perspective, chronological age is less important than it used to be.

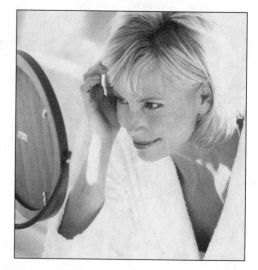

Still, it's nice to think that our outsides communicate how good we feel *inside*. Taking care of your skin the natural way can get that message out.

Skin Care from A to Z

What's the fundamental rule of natural skin care? Stop punishing your skin by exposing it to the things that cause aging. Here's a list of skin's most important enemies and how to avoid them, courtesy of Gloria Graham, M.D., a dermatologist in Morehead City, North Carolina.

• Avoid direct exposure to sunlight whenever possible. By one estimate, at least 80 percent of all visible skin aging results from a lifetime of repeated sun exposure. "To get some idea of the effects of sun exposure, take a look at the skin on your breasts or abdomen," Dr. Graham says. "That's how your skin would look now if you had protected it."

• Keep your weight stable. Repeatedly losing and gaining causes skin to sag.

• Remove makeup thoroughly. Avoid cosmetics that clog the skin's hair follicles, causing blemishes. Look for products labeled nonacnegenic (won't provoke acne) and noncomedogenic (won't provoke blackheads and whiteheads).

• Use a cleansing sponge (like a loofah or Buf-Puf) to get rid of dead skin cells and open the skin's hair follicles. Keep the sponge away from the delicate area around your eyes.

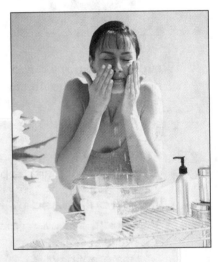

Wrinkle Rehab

More than good scents, pure essential oils can help smooth and plump wrinkled skin, says Amanda McQuade Crawford, a practicing herbalist in Ojai, California, and author of *Herbal Remedies for Women*.

Start with an ounce of honey or a cup of cooled herbal tea. (Chamomile tea soothes the skin, while nettle tea nourishes it, McQuade Crawford says.) Then add a drop or two of sandalwood, lavender, clary sage, or chamomile essential oil, she suggests. For oily skin, try a citrus variety such as lemon or tangerine. For dry skin, make it rose. "This helps moisturize and brings blood flow to the surface of the skin. And remember, less is more. You only need a few drops of essential oil."

Smoothed on your skin several times a week as a skin treatment, this formula can begin to improve the look of wrinkled skin in 6 to 8 weeks, says McQuade Crawford. Remember to keep essential oils and formulas that contain them away from your eyes and mouth.

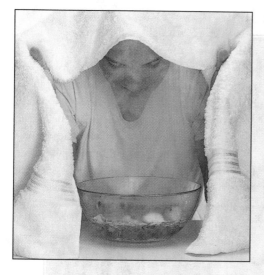

Steam Therapy

A weekly or monthly facial steam is not only a good way to clean your pores, it's a lovely time to relax and pamper yourself," says Donna Bryant, an herbalist in Pembroke, New Hampshire, who teaches at Sage Mountain herbal education center in East Barre, Vermont. "You'll quickly discover that herbs are good for your spirit as well as for your skin." The herbs can be customized for your skin type.

For normal to dry skin: Bryant suggests combining two parts calendula flowers, two parts borage, one part lavender, one part chamomile, one part roses, and one-half part fennel seeds. "These herbs help to soften dry, rough skin," she says.

For oily skin: Try two parts comfrey, two parts calendula, two parts witch hazel, one part yarrow, and one part rosemary. "These are soothing and astringent herbs that will help ease oil production," notes Bryant. Add one part peppermint for a refreshing zing.

What You'll Need

Assemble the following materials for your steam facial.

- Teakettle
- Heatproof bowl
- Fresh or dried herbs chosen for your specific skin type
- Large towel

Heat it up. Place 3 cups of water in a teakettle and bring it to a boil, then carefully pour the steaming water into a heatproof bowl. Add about a cup of your herb blend.

Steam away. Drape a large towel over your head and lean over the bowl close enough to feel the steam (about 12 inches away), but not so close that it burns. "You simply want to build up a rolling sweat on your skin," says Bryant. Steam for 5 to 20 minutes, then pat your face dry. Follow with a mask for more cleansing or with a toner and moisturizer.

Those are the basics. Now take the next step. Certain nutritional supplements can also help keep your skin healthy and young-looking. Try the following nutrition prescription, suggests Dr. Graham.

• 5,000 international units (IU) of vitamin A daily, if you are not getting enough from foods. A deficiency of vitamin A can leave skin rough and scaly.

• 500 milligrams of vitamin C daily. Vitamin C supports the formation of collagen, the connective tissue that gives skin its structure and tone.

• 400 IU of vitamin E daily. Vitamin E is an antioxidant that helps protect the skin against sun damage. If you are considering taking this amount, discuss it with your doctor first. One study using low-dose supplements showed increased risk of hemorrhagic stroke.

• 200 micrograms of selenium daily. In studies, people with low levels of selenium appear most prone to skin cancer.

Knowing the fundamental rules of good skin care doesn't mean you'll have the skin of a movie star every day of the week. Mere mortals are not so lucky. The following collection of natural remedies, all recommended by experts, will help you address inevitable chinks in your epidermal armor.

Age Spots

Age spots have nothing to do with age. Rather, these flat, brown patches result from overexposure to the sun. Now they can be prevented with the help of sunscreen, but truly protective sunscreen products didn't appear on the market until

Black and White

For sun safety, basic black is better. Dark-colored clothing will absorb ultraviolet rays, preventing them from reaching your skin, according to Rodney Basler, M.D., assistant professor of internal medicine at the University of Nebraska Medical Center in Lincoln.

"We used to think that white clothing was the best outerwear because it would reflect sunlight, but in fact, the sun's rays penetrate light-colored clothes," says Dr. Basler. He first discovered this upon observing the striped tan that his little girl had developed after a day at the beach in a black-and-white-striped bathing suit.

the early 1980s. So anyone born before then is likely to develop age spots.

Here are several steps you can take to fade existing spots and discourage new spots from forming.

Make 'em fade. Apply a fade cream that contains 2 percent hydroquinone. It will help diminish age spots, although they won't disappear completely. Follow the label directions carefully. If left on too long, fade creams can irritate the skin.

Discover AHAs. To lighten age spots and even out skin tone, apply a cream or lotion that contains alpha hydroxy acids (AHAs). These natural acids strip away dead skin cells and prompt the growth of fresh, new cells. Choose a 5 percent AHA preparation and follow the label instructions, being careful not to get the cream or lotion near your eyes. You may experience some tingling when you first apply it, but it should subside within a few minutes.

Wash your hands after handling food. Celery, limes, and other foods contain psoralens, chemicals that can cause a sunburnlike reaction in the skin when exposed to sunlight. The affected skin eventually blisters and heals with hyperpigmentation (darker skin), which can persist for weeks to months.

Monitor medicines. Certain drugs make your skin more sensitive to sunlight, so you are more likely to develop age spots. Among the offenders: Retin-A, used for acne and wrinkles; antibiotics such as tetracycline; and blood pressure and diabetes medications.

Crow's-Feet

Here's one of the clearer examples of the toll that the sun can take on your skin. Squint long and often enough, and the temporary wrinkle patterns that form at the corners of your eyes will eventually become permanent. Smoking only adds to the problem. In addition to wearing hats and sunscreen, keep crow's-feet at a minimum with the following natural remedies.

Remoisturize with cocoa. Keep the area around your eyes moist by applying skin lotions and cosmetics daily that are enriched with cocoa butter. Cocoa contains emollients that help prevent dryness, while moisturizing and softening the skin. Coconut oil is a similar tropical emollient that offers the same benefits.

Pat on papaya. To loosen and remove old, sun-wrinkled cells on the skin's surface, make a homemade facial peel using papaya and fresh

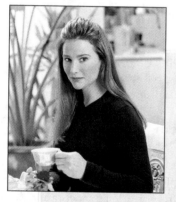

HEALING SPOTLIGHT
Keely Shaye Smith

Keely Shaye Smith has an active life as a broadcast journalist and avid gardener. She also finds time to spend with actor Pierce Brosnan, father of her child and love of her life. Smith attributes her good health and radiant skin in part to the many natural tonics she uses, from ginseng to garlic. Here she explains why the healing plant aloe vera is "a staple" in her house.

"I break open the leaves of the plant and use the wonderful gel on my skin every morning. It can be used on any kind of skin abrasion, insect bites. . . . It's also good for the scalp.

"Aloe vera also helps my hands stay soft—but if you look at my hands you can tell I'm a real gardener at home by these calluses!"

pineapple juice. The peel will reveal a layer of smooth, fresher-looking skin.

Purchase a papaya in the produce section of your super-market. It doesn't have to be ripe to work. At home, mash ¼ cup of pulp. To enhance its skin-peeling properties, add 1 teaspoon of fresh pineapple juice to the mashed pulp. Apply this mixture to the wrinkled skin around your eyes. Be careful not to get the pulp in your eyes. (If you do, rinse im-mediately with cool water.) You can also spread it on your entire face and neck. Leave the pulp on your skin for 10 to 15 minutes, then rinse with luke-warm water. It may sting slightly, but that's a sign that it's working. Repeat twice a week.

Rose hips to the rescue. Strong rose hip tea also works as a mild facial peel. The ascorbic acid in this herb peels away the upper layers of skin cells. To make a rose hip peel, put 1 tablespoon of dried rose hips in ½ cup of boiling water. Steep for 15 minutes, then cool. Using your fingers, pat the cooled tea on the skin over your crow's-feet. Leave it on for 5 minutes, then rinse with tepid water. Finish the treatment by applying a light application of olive oil to moisturize your skin.

‖ Dry ‖ Skin

Skin naturally loses some water to the envi-ronment through evaporation. But if your skin

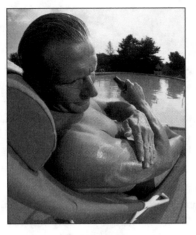

"A healthy tan is an oxymoron."
—John DiGiovanna, M.D., director of dermatopharma-cology at Brown University School of Medicine in Providence, Rhode Island

has trouble retaining water, it will be prone to dryness. Chapped, cracking skin won't protect you from viruses and infections as well as it should. So keeping it hydrated is essential. It is also quite easy to do, as these tips demonstrate.

Moisturize with some milk. Pour cold milk into a bowl or basin, then dip a washcloth or a piece of gauze in the milk and hold it against the affected skin for 5 minutes. Milk soothes dry skin and has anti-inflammatory properties to relieve itching.

Moisturize with a little mineral oil. Plain old mineral oil traps mois-ture in the skin, helping it stay hydrated.

Rehydrate with this slippery bedtime ritual. Before going to bed, soak in a lukewarm bath almost to the point where your fingertips shrivel like prunes—your skin will be fully hydrated. Get out of the tub, pat yourself semi-dry, and apply a thick layer of solid shortening to the affected skin. Slip into an old pair of pajamas and climb into bed. (Since the shortening is messy, you may want to use old bedsheets, too.) Your skin will feel and look much better by morning.

Cleanse gently. For your daily shower or bath, use lukewarm water and a very mild soap. If your skin is extremely dry, avoid strong antibacterial soaps, which tend to dry skin out even more.

Oily Skin

Everyone's skin has a coating of oil, or sebum, to keep out dirt and make skin soft and supple. Sometimes, the oil becomes too thick, thanks to overproductive sebaceous glands. The skin feels greasy, looks shiny, and is more prone to breakouts.

Oily skin tends to be hereditary. It is especially common among dark-haired women, who naturally have thicker skin and more sebaceous glands than blonde-haired women.

Like dry skin, oily skin becomes a problem only when it isn't properly cared for. You can minimize the sheen and reduce the likelihood of breakouts by following this advice.

Buy the right bar. To wash your face, use a soap made with glycerin, cucumber, witch hazel, or citrus acids. These natural ingredients keep oily skin healthy. Soaps made with these natural ingredients can be found in drugstores or bath-and-beauty shops. Avoid superfatted soaps, which are intended to moisturize as they clean. They only add oil to the skin.

Lather up less. Washing your face too often may stimulate your skin to produce *more* oil. Limit yourself to three times a day, tops.

Try a natural toner. After washing your face, use a cotton ball to apply witch hazel.

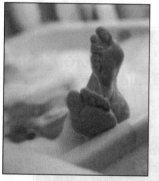

Low-Tech Foot Relief

Where can you get soft, smooth feet? Between a rock and a hard place. Underneath those rough spots and hard calluses lies smooth skin just waiting to be exposed. And the easiest way to do that is with the lowly, low-tech pumice stone, available at drugstores or discount stores.

Look for a hand-size stone that's easy to grip. Use the stone firmly but gently (never break the skin) to exfoliate feet, advises Andrea Carcchiolo, M.D., professor of orthopedic surgery at the University of California, Los Angeles. An important caveat: Don't pumice too often or too harshly. The stone eliminates calluses by using friction, the same thing that causes the problem. If you overpumice your feet, you may eventually cause more rough skin to build up. Use the stone a maximum of once a week.

Pumice maintenance is easy. Treat it like your toothbrush: Have your own personal pumice stone, rinse after each use, and allow to air dry. Unlike your toothbrush, however, a pumice will last for years. "When it doesn't smooth your skin any longer, you know it's time to get a new one," says Dr. Carcchiolo.

A mild astringent, witch hazel will clean soap residues from your skin and reduce the amount of oil on your skin.

Fight oil with (essential) oil. Add two drops of lemongrass essential oil to ½ ounce of a carrier oil such as apricot kernel, flaxseed, or hazelnut (available in most health food stores). After every cleansing, gently apply the mixture to your face with a cotton ball or with your clean fingers. Lemongrass helps degrease the skin and regulates overactive sebaceous glands. You may use it on a daily basis if necessary. But keep it away from your eyes.

Puffy Eyes

Crying, too little sleep, simple aging, water retention, salty foods—all can leave you with bags under your eyes. Instead of hiding them with makeup, let nature's remedies do the job.

Make a cold fennel compress. Fennel tea has a nice aroma and a soothing, moisturizing effect on your eyes. To make a 4-day supply of tea, pour a cup of boiling water over 2 teaspoons of fennel seeds and cover. Let the mixture steep, then put the whole pot in the refrigerator overnight, leaving the seeds in. In the morning, strain the cooled tea. Soak the tea in beautician's cotton (available at beauty supply stores) or paper towels, lie down with your head elevated on a pillow, and cover your closed eyes with the patches. Soak for 10 to 15 minutes, rewetting the patches whenever they warm up.

Drink dandelion tea. Dandelion is a cleansing diuretic that flushes out excess fluid accumulation. To make dandelion tea, use 1 teaspoon of dried dandelion leaf and 1 teaspoon of root per cup of boiling water. Steep in a

Allergy Alert

They may be found in health food stores, but they're not without side effects: Skin care products containing herbs such as cinnamon, vanilla, oil of clove, or laurel oil can trigger powerful allergic reactions in some people, says Arnold Schroeter, M.D., chair of the dermatology department at the Mayo Clinic in Rochester, Minnesota. Even tea tree oil—used on everything from burns to blemishes to dry scalp—may cause contact dermatitis, says Dr. Schroeter.

To avoid an uncomfortable reaction, do a trial application. Rub the ointment or oil on your inner forearm near your elbow two or three times a day for a couple of days. That way, if you get a reaction, it's limited to one spot, not your whole face or body. People who tend to be particularly hypersensitive to herbal products are those with fair, dry, or irritable skin.

teapot or covered container for 10 minutes, then strain. Drink three cups a day until symptoms improve.

Spider Veins

At least 40 percent of women develop spider veins—networks of tiny red, blue, or purple blood vessels that appear on the upper thighs, behind the knees, and on the feet. They can be caused by a superficial injury, anything from being hit by a tennis ball to being jumped on by a pet. They are also quite common during pregnancy: Nearly two-thirds of moms-to-be get them.

Spider veins may be unsightly, but they seldom cause the pain and swelling associated with varicose veins. Still, most women who have them would just as soon see them disappear. You can have them removed by laser or injection. If you prefer to go the natural route, doctors suggest these strategies.

Have a bowl of berries. Fruits like blueberries, blackberries, cherries, and raspberries supply bioflavonoids, natural compounds that help strengthen blood vessels. The darker the fruit, the more bioflavonoids it contains.

Don't peel away the pith. Pith, the white membrane in citrus fruits such as oranges and grapefruit, also provides a healthy dose of bioflavonoids.

Go for ginkgo. The herb ginkgo helps strengthen the tissues that form vein walls. You can buy ginkgo supplements in health food stores. Look for a 50:1 extract, which will be specified on the label. Take 40 milligrams three times a day until spider veins are diminished.

Varicose Veins

Veins become varicose, or swollen, when the valves lining the vein walls fail to do their job. Normally, these valves prevent blood from

> **NATURAL**FACT
>
> Adding a half-cup of baking soda to warm bath water naturally cleanses your skin and leaves you feeling silky smooth all over.

flowing backward when it is making a return trip to the heart. A valve opens, the blood goes through, and the valve closes. But if that valve malfunctions, it allows the blood to reverse direction and pool in the vein. Eventually, the pressure created by the pooled blood stretches the vein wall. That's when the vein becomes visible on the surface of the skin.

Why do some women get varicose veins while others don't? Genetics, mostly. If your mother (or father) has varicose veins, you are likely to have them, too. Your risk increases if you are overweight or you stand for 6 or more hours a day.

Pregnancy can also contribute to the development of varicose veins, for a couple of reasons. First, the hormonal changes that occur during pregnancy allow the veins to stretch to accommodate extra bloodflow. Second, the weight of the fetus can interfere with bloodflow and put greater pressure on the leg veins, especially during the third trimester.

For the most part, varicose veins are viewed as a cosmetic problem. But they can produce a variety of physical symptoms, too, including throbbing pain, burning or itchy skin, and swollen legs and feet.

Fortunately, you don't have to put up with unsightly veins that make your legs feel tired and heavy. These strategies can minimize your discomfort and keep varicose veins from worsening.

Comfort with a compress. Put ½ to 1 cup of distilled witch hazel in a bowl and refrigerate it for at least 1 hour. Then add six drops of cypress essential oil, one drop of lemon essential oil, and one drop of bergamot essential oil. Soak a cloth in the witch hazel solution, then lay the cloth over the varicose vein for 15 minutes. While applying the compress, elevate your feet on a few pillows to support circulation. Both the witch hazel and the essential oils have an astringent effect—they shrink small blood vessels near the surface of the skin, temporarily reducing swelling.

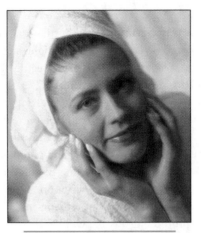

Skin—like the rest of the body—has the capacity to repair itself.

Eye aescin. In one study, taking 50 milligrams of aescin (the extract from the dried seeds of the horse chestnut plant) twice a day for 12 weeks reduced the lower-leg swelling associated with varicose veins by 25 percent. Aescin also appears to strengthen blood vessel walls, helping to prevent veins from softening and bulging. Aescin is available at health food stores.

Get your fill of roughage. Every day, eat at least 25 grams (the Daily Value) of fiber. A fiber-rich diet featuring whole grains, fruits, and vegetables helps prevent constipation by making stool easier to pass. If you must strain to move your bowels, you create pressure in your abdomen that can block the flow of blood to your legs. Over time, the increased pressure may weaken the walls of the veins in your legs.

Stock up on C. Your body uses vitamin C to build collagen and elastin, connective tissues that help strengthen vein walls. Take 500 milligrams twice a day.

Move your legs. Even while you are sitting, you can do simple exercises to keep the blood in your legs circulating. Here's one to try. Flex your feet, lifting your toes while keeping your heels down, as though you are pumping a piano pedal. Continue for a minute or two, then repeat every hour.

‖ Wrinkles

We've already said it, but it's worth saying again: Unprotected sun exposure is the leading cause of wrinkles. It wreaks havoc on the skin by breaking down collagen and elastin, two connective tissues that give skin its structure and tone.

Fortunately, skin—like the rest of the body—has the capacity to repair itself. You can take steps to diminish existing wrinkles and discourage new ones from appearing. Here's what dermatologists recommend.

Say yes to AHAs. AHAs fight wrinkles in two ways. First, they loosen and remove old, wrinkled cells to uncover the young, fresh cells underneath. Second, they plump the skin's surface—in essence, filling in the "dents" that you see as wrinkles. Use an 8 percent AHA preparation on your face and neck twice a day—once in the morning and once at night. For the sensitive area around the eyes, use a fragrance-free 5 percent AHA eye cream and avoid getting it into your eyes or on your eyelashes. If you do, thoroughly rinse the affected eye with cold water.

Moisturize in the morning. Plumping up your skin with moisturizer can help hide existing wrinkles. But most women apply moisturizer before they go to bed, so their appearance is improved for only 4 to 6 hours while they sleep. You are better off moisturizing first thing in the morning.

Smooth on topical vitamin C. Unlike AHAs, which reverse skin damage by speeding up the exfoliation process, vitamin C may help prevent damage in the first place. As an antioxidant, vitamin C protects against wrinkles by fighting off free radicals, unstable molecules that form when the skin is exposed to sunlight and ultraviolet radiation and that harm healthy cells and contribute to skin damage.

Applying vitamin C directly to your skin can help prevent depletion of the nutrient when you spend a lot of time in the sun. One topical vitamin C product is Cellex-C, a 10 percent vitamin C solution that's available without a prescription from dermatologists and licensed aestheticians. The solution provides your skin with 20 times the vitamin C that you would get from your diet.

NATURAL HEALING THROUGH HISTORY

Cleopatra: Secrets of an Ageless Beauty Queen

Judging from the profile that appeared on the coins she commissioned, Cleopatra's features weren't all that attractive, at least not by today's standards. Even so, her reputation as the original femme fatale suggests an extraordinary allure.

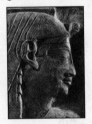

Cleopatra reigned as queen of Egypt from 51 to 30 B.C. Historians say that her rule was characterized by ruthless ambition and manipulation—but then, most historians are men.

However you describe her tactics, for an extraordinary period she managed, against great odds, to maintain her country's independence from Roman rule—and her own power on the Egyptian throne.

The Greek historian Dio Cassius called her "brilliant to look upon, with the power to subjugate everyone." Another ancient biographer, Plutarch, wrote that she had a voice like "an instrument of many strings," with which she could speak at least seven languages and a thousand "sorts of flattery." Certainly, she was skilled at flattering herself. She is said to have written a book on cosmetics that was divided into sections on foot, hand, skin, hair, and tooth care. Although the original has been lost, portions of her wisdom have supposedly been passed down through the ages, with many subsequent beauty experts claiming to have come into possession of her secrets. Her repertoire is said to have included clay from the Nile River, minerals and mud from around the Dead Sea, buttermilk-and-aloe-vera baths, egg masks, berry juices, beeswax, and almond oil. It's even been rumored that she wore a magnet on her forehead to help maintain her youthful beauty.

Whether it was through her beauty, her charisma, or both, Cleopatra managed to enchant the most powerful men of her day, including Julius Caesar of Rome and his leading general, Marc Antony. Legend has it that she sailed to meet Antony in a magnificently gilded river barge with silver oars and purple sails drenched in jasmine. Maidens dressed as sea nymphs and servant boys dressed as cupids attended her on the journey. Cleopatra herself was arrayed as Venus, the goddess of love. Not surprisingly, Antony is said to have fallen for her at first sight.

Cleopatra's reign came to an end when Caesar's heir, Octavian, triumphed over Antony and bore down upon Egypt. The queen is said to have committed suicide by allowing herself to be bitten by an asp, a symbol of divine royalty. Death by snakebite was thought to secure immortality, and perhaps it has for Cleopatra. The legend of this ancient enchantress still lives on today.

Chapter 5

Make Your Hair a Natural Wonder

Tame your hair-abuse problem—undo the damage, naturally

Hair. It can be our crowning glory or an exasperating embarrassment. A halo of health and beauty, or a tangled, misbegotten mess.

If it's less often glory and more often mess, usually we can only blame ourselves. A lifetime of straightening, teasing, rolling, ironing, primping, coloring, and frizzing takes a toll. There's also the problem of drought: as you age, your hair naturally dries out.

What to do?

First, you can decide to stop the cruel and unusual hair punishment. The less you primp, iron, tease, and roll now, the healthier your hair will be in the long run.

Second, you can send your hair to nature's rehab.

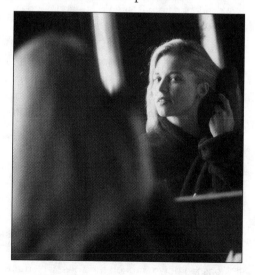

Dry Hair

In healthy hair, the cells that make up each strand's outer layer, called the cuticle, overlap like shingles on a roof. If the cells are roughed up or chipped away, the strand loses moisture and doesn't reflect light as it should. So hair not only feels dry, but looks dry, too.

What causes hair cells to get out of line? Perhaps the chief offender is overprocessing—coloring, perming, and straightening. Exposure to sun and chlorine, misuse and overuse of styling implements such as blow-dryers and curling irons, and even poorly made brushes and combs can leave hair parched, dull, and coarse to the touch.

With a few simple changes in your hair-care routine, experts say, you can repair the damage that leads to dry hair.

Be picky about shampoo. Look for a shampoo that contains aloe, glycerin, honey, amino acids, or natural oils. All of these substances moisturize hair.

It Goes to Your Head

Back in the 1950s, teenage girls rinsed their hair with beer to make it shine. And who knows where they got the idea. Maybe a chemistry teacher—there seems to be something to it.

One of the main reasons why your hair loses its shine is because of damage to the outer layer of the hair shaft called the cuticle. The cuticle is lined with scales that resemble shingles on a rooftop. When the scales lay smooth on the shaft, they reflect light. Because of sun exposure, overbrushing, and chemical assaults on your hair, the shingles become loose and curl upward, making hair look dull.

The protein found in beer can fill in the irregular surface between the scales of the cuticle, causing a smoother appearance and more shine, says Leslie Baumann, M.D., director and assistant professor of cosmetic dermatology at the University of Miami. For the best results, soak your hair thoroughly with the beer, then rinse. Be sure to use beer that's fresh and still foaming, because the proteins necessary to make the head on the beer are the same ones that add shine to hair. Stale beer has no head because these proteins have already been broken down. And just as with any conditioner, beer's shining effect only lasts until the next washing.

Moisturize with essential oils. If you can't find a commercial conditioner that you like, make your own instead. Add six drops each of lavender, bay, and sandalwood essential oils (available in health food stores) to 6 ounces of warm sesame or soy oil. Part your hair into 1-inch sections and apply the oil blend to your scalp with a wad of cotton. Wrap your head in a towel and wait 15 minutes. Then uncover your hair and shampoo twice.

Dry wisely. Whenever possible, use only a towel to pat or gently squeeze water from your hair. If you must use a blow-dryer, apply a thermal styling conditioner to protect your hair. Set the dryer on high to remove residual water, then switch to low for styling. Hold the dryer at least 6 to 8 inches from your hair at all times.

Save with sandalwood. Brittle, fly-away ends can be restored with a few drops of sandalwood oil. Mix the sandalwood in a carrier oil such as olive or jojoba. Rub it on your palms, then across the ends of your hair.

Mellow with marshmallow. Marshmallow root has a natural moisturizing quality that can make a hair-pleasing herbal rinse. To make, add 2 teaspoons of dried marshmallow root to a cup of boiling water, strain, and cool in the refrigerator.

Graying Hair

If you wonder when your hair will start turning gray (if it hasn't already), take a look at mom and dad. Graying is hereditary, and there's no avoiding it. Everyone eventually goes gray as individual hair follicles stop producing pigment.

Surprisingly, only about one-third of all women opt for the cover-up. The rest let nature make the choice. But even Mother

Survival of the Blondest

Why does gray hair supposedly look "distinguished" on men but not on women? Scientists believe that the answer goes back to the reproductive preferences of the Stone Age.

Our male ancestors chose mates whose physical appearance suggested that they were fertile and would bear healthy offspring. Gray locks on a woman were a physical cue that her youth—more specifically, her fertility—had passed.

To our foremothers, on the other hand, gray hair on a potential mate was a plus. Those steely locks meant that he had resources, power, and status—the kinds of things that would enable him to help protect their babies.

Somewhere in the small Stone Age part of our brains, those ancient signals are still being irresistibly transmitted, and a part of us still listens.

Nature has some secrets to help give gray hair a youthful sheen.

Rinse with sage or rosemary. To gently darken brown or black hair that's showing signs of gray, use a rinse made from sage or rosemary. Add between 2 teaspoons and 1 tablespoon of either dried herb to a cup of boiling water. Let the liquid cool to a comfortable temperature, strain out the herb, and pour the liquid over your hair after shampooing. Don't rinse it out. Repeat each time you wash your hair, until you've covered the gray.

Add nettle and walnut to the mix. For auburn, brown, or medium to dark gray hair, use a coloring made with nettle and black walnut hulls (available at health food stores or through mail-order catalogs). To prepare the coloring, boil 8 cups of water and add ¼ cup each of dried sage, rosemary, and nettle; ½ cup of black walnut hulls; and two black tea bags. Allow the mixture to steep for 3 hours, then strain out the herbs and walnut hulls and add 2 teaspoons of sweet almond or olive oil. Keep the mixture refrigerated until you're ready to use it. After you wash and rinse your hair, slip on a pair of rubber gloves and work ½ cup of the mixture through your hair, being careful not to get it on your forehead, neck, and temples. Wait a minute or so before towel drying your hair. (Use a dark towel so the stains won't show.)

Oily Hair

The term *oily hair* is something of a misnomer. The oil comes not from your hair but from your scalp.

Your scalp, like the rest of your skin, has sebaceous glands. They secrete sebum, a mixture of fatty acids that keeps your scalp from drying out. In some people, the sebaceous glands churn out so much sebum that each hair shaft becomes slickly coated

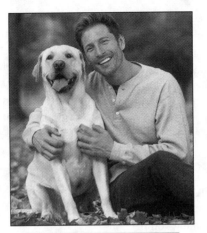

"He may have hair upon his chest but, sister, so has Lassie."

—"I Hate Men"

by Cole Porter

and weighted down. Hair appears greasy, flat, and lifeless.

Sebum production is regulated by hormones. It shifts into overdrive during puberty, pregnancy, and menopause—times of significant hormonal changes. It's also accelerated by oral contraceptives that contain mostly androgen, a male sex hormone.

Women who have oily hair often find that the problem literally dries up after they go through menopause, when their hormone levels decline. In the meantime, you can control greasiness by following this advice.

Wash in the A.M. You work up a sweat while you sleep. So by morning, even hair shampooed just before bedtime looks oily and matted.

Stir up your own shampoo. Add four drops of rosemary essential oil and four drops of lavender essential oil to 2 ounces of any unscented shampoo. Shake to mix well, then use a quarter-size dollop to wash your hair. Rosemary and lavender tone your scalp and add shine. The essential oils are available in health food stores and bath-and-beauty shops.

Rinse with vinegar. Vinegar reduces soap and hard-water residues to make your hair soft and shiny. Mix 1 cup of vinegar with 1 cup of water, then pour the solution over your hair as your final rinse. Vinegar's aroma quickly fades, so you won't smell like a salad.

Finish with an herbal rinse. To complete your hair-washing regimen, herbalists suggest this oil-fighting herbal rinse: Pour 1 pint of boiling water over 1 teaspoon each of the dried herbs burdock root, calendula flowers, chamomile flowers, lavender flowers, lemongrass, and sage leaves. Steep for about 30 minutes. Strain and add 1 tablespoon of vinegar. Pour this herbal mix over your scalp and hair as a final rinse after shampooing. For best results, don't rinse it out. The herbs discourage excess oil production, while the vinegar helps prevent dandruff.

Curtail conditioning. Most conditioners and styling products contain ingredients that weigh hair down, the last thing you need if your hair is oily. If you have an oily scalp and fine hair, apply conditioner only to the ends of your hair, not to your scalp.

Cut back on brushing. The more you brush, the more you spread oil from your scalp to your hair. So keep brushing to a minimum; brush just to keep your hair in place.

Thinning Hair

Everyone sheds between 50 and 100 hairs per day. The average hair has a life span of 3 to 6 years, entering a resting stage of about 3 months before falling out. Then a new hair sprouts in its place from the same root.

Sometimes, though, the hair-growth cycle gets messed up, causing hundreds of hairs to fall out per day. In women, hormonal changes brought on by pregnancy, menopause, and the use of oral contraceptives can alter hair-growing conditions. So can rapid weight loss, iron deficiency, serious illness, and extreme physical stress (such as childbirth). Women can also have a genetic predisposition to hair loss, just as men do.

If you seem to be losing more hair than normal, see your doctor. She can examine you for

Hair Dye Warning

Be careful of progressive hair dyes. Those that contain an ingredient called lead acetate can contain up to 10 times the amount of lead allowed in house paint—a lead source that remains a major health hazard. Users can spread significant amounts of lead to their hands, combs, blow-dryers, even telephones. Check the label: If lead acetate is not listed, then your hair dye is okay.

an underlying medical problem and prescribe proper treatment. Then use these measures to care for your remaining hair and discourage more loss.

Baby your mane. Wash your hair with a baby shampoo, lathering up only once and rubbing your scalp gently. After rinsing, spray your hair with a detangling conditioner.

Pull the plug. Allow your hair to dry naturally whenever possible. If you must use a blow-dryer, set it on low.

Wait while wet. Wait until your hair is completely dry before combing or brushing. Otherwise, it can stretch and break. And never tease your hair, which also causes breakage.

Mine for iron. Iron deficiency can contribute to hair loss, so eat one or two servings of iron-rich foods every day. Good sources of the mineral include lean red meat, Cream of Wheat cereal, tofu, and broccoli.

Put protein on your plate. Without adequate protein, your body can't make new hair to replace what has fallen out. So eat two 3- to 4-ounce servings of chicken, fish, or other lean protein every day.

NATURAL HEALING IN THE FUTURE

Living to 120—Or Longer

Timothy J. Smith, M.D., author of *Renewal: The Anti-Aging Revolution*, is at the forefront of the rapidly growing field of anti-aging medicine. Here, he talks about where the anti-aging revolution is today and where it will be going in the future.

Q: What is the status of anti-aging medicine right now?

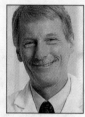

A: There are thousands of doctors and researchers involved in the field, and they are focusing on many different areas. There's brain fitness, age-reversing dermatology, anti-aging dentistry, phytohormones, antioxidant therapies, gene therapy, restoration of youthful metabolism. The list goes on. Most doctors see this work as an outgrowth of mainstream medicine. For me, it was more a realization that if you create harmony and balance in the body, you're also going to dramatically slow down the aging process. That's why I think that the basics of diet and supplements and exercise are so important, as opposed to just focusing on the high-tech stuff.

Q: But the high-tech stuff is pretty mind-blowing, isn't it?

A: Well, you can't really talk about anti-aging without mentioning genetic engi-

neering. It's not something that people can actually use at this point, but it holds the biggest hope for major breakthroughs. You can fiddle with things like hormone supplements and get closer to achieving a lifespan of 120 years; but to go beyond that is going to require altering genes. And that's going to happen. No question.

Q: What specifically do you expect to see developed?

A: The most exciting genetic research has to do with telomeres. Those are the little protein caps on the ends of chromosomes that protect them. They wear out gradually with age and when that happens, their cells die. Recent research has found that when you replace telomerase, it creates an immortal cell. It's definitely the hottest thing on the horizon right now for genetically changing our aging.

Q: Would it stop you from getting diseases?

A: It would slow them down. But even when we can program cells not to die any more, we'll still be stuck with the problem of free radicals, those unstable particles that careen around damaging healthy cells and setting the stage for degenerative diseases. So taking antioxidants and eating a plant-based diet in order to minimize free radical production is still going to be critical to living a long time.

One supplement can help protect you from diabetes, heart disease, high blood pressure, osteoporosis, and migraines.

Part Three

Healing with
Vitamins

*Vitamin and mineral supplements can build your body's
natural defenses against illness, boost energy, and make you feel great.*

Chapter 6

Test Your Vitamin and Supplement I.Q.

Yes, you can get natural nutrients in a pill, but do you know what to look for?

Vitamin and mineral choices used to be so simple: Wilma or Fred? Barney or Dino? Now every time you go into a drugstore, you're faced with a supplements section the size of an airplane hangar.

There's a lot in those endless rows of bottles that can give you more energy, help you get sick less often, and live longer. The problem is that to get those benefits, it really helps to know a little bit about things that seem designed to make your eyes glaze over instantly. Things like RDA. Milligrams. The difference between B_6 and B_{12}.

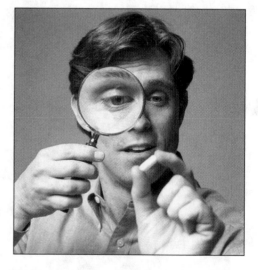

Perhaps you're already an ace at this stuff. Perhaps not. Find out by taking our vitamin-and-mineral quiz.

Answers are on page 50.

The Questions, Please

1. Is it okay for you to take your kid's chewable vitamin?

a. No, because children's vitamins have far fewer vitamins and minerals than adult versions

b. Yes, because I probably need the same nutrients as my child

c. No, because kids' vitamins have more vitamins and minerals than adults' to help their growing bodies

2. You've just been to a company picnic where you indulged in more drinking than you normally do. Drinking causes you to lose what?

a. Sodium

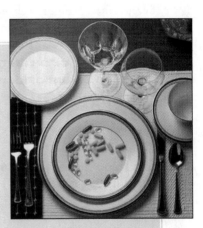

A Question of Timing

When is the best time to take your vitamins? The short answer is: whenever you're most likely to remember to take them. Consistency is more important than time of day.

That said, here is how to get the biggest possible payoff from the supplements you take, according to Holly McCord, R.D., *Prevention* magazine's nutrition editor.

Multis. Take with a meal, and make sure the meal includes at least a little fat (about 5 grams, or the amount in 1 teaspoon of margarine) to help you absorb fat-soluble vitamins A, D, E, and K. Drink some fluid to help multis dissolve.

Vitamin E. Take with a meal or snack with a little fat, as with multis.

Vitamin C. Take half of your daily dose at breakfast and half at dinner to keep blood levels high throughout the day.

Calcium. Take 500 milligrams or less at a time to maximize absorption. Take calcium carbonate with a meal or snack for best absorption; calcium citrate may be taken between meals. Cereals high in wheat bran reduce calcium absorption. A calcium supplement before bedtime may limit calcium loss from your bones while you sleep.

Iron. Taking iron supplements or a multi with iron at the same time as calcium supplements will reduce iron absorption. If iron is a concern, take calcium supplements at a different time. (But don't take iron supplements unless you are diagnosed with iron deficiency.)

b. Potassium

c. B vitamins, particularly thiamin

d. Your balance

3. Why were British sailors called limeys?

a. Because their faces turned the color of limes when they got seasick

b. Because someone once told them to eat citrus fruits, such as limes, to combat scurvy

c. Because their uniforms were lime green

d. Because French sailors were called lemonheads

4. Which mineral joins vitamins A, C, and E as an antioxidant?

a. Selenium

b. Magnesium

c. Iron

d. Chromium

5. Which mineral transports oxygen in the blood?

a. Chromium

b. Zinc

c. Sulfur

d. Iron

6. What's the difference between vitamins and minerals?

a. Vitamin are needed in larger amounts

b. Vitamins come from organic things, minerals come from nonorganic things

c. Vitamins don't have names, just letters and numbers

d. All of the above

Uncle Sam's Advice

At the start of World War II, the U.S. government found that many men who wanted to enlist in the military had vitamin and mineral deficiencies that made them vulnerable to disease. That discovery prompted the government to begin issuing its list of Recommended Dietary Allowances (RDAs) in 1943. About 50 years later, a simplified version of these allowances was unveiled under the name Daily Values (DV).

7. Is beta-carotene added to processed food for coloring?

a. Yes, because it's a pigment that can make foods more yellow-orange

b. No, because it's found in green, leafy vegetables

8. Which diseases are caused by vitamin or mineral deficiencies?

a. Pellagra

b. Beriberi

c. Cretinism

d. Goiter

e. Night blindness

f. All of the above

Correct answers: 1. b; 2. c.; 3. b.; 4. a.; 5. d.; 6. b.; 7. a.; 8. f.

Chapter 7

Vitamins and Supplements 2000

A guide to what's hot, what's great, and what you can do without

Frankly, there are times when we find supplements as confusing as anybody else does, but we've tried to remedy that. We hunted down experts, reviewed studies, and got the goods on many of the nutrients and other nonherbal supplements you may have heard about.

The first thing we'd recommend is picking up a good multivitamin/mineral supplement, plus separate supplements of vitamins C and E, and calcium. (See "Everyday Supplements" on page 58 for specifics.) Even if you eat well and exercise, you're unlikely to get optimum levels of all the essential nutrients from food alone. Supplements, therefore, make sense.

Here's what to look for in your store's vitamin section.

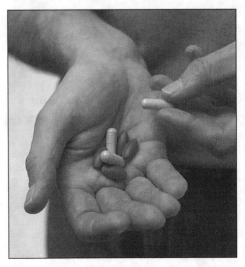

Special Bonus!

At-a-Glance Vitamin and Mineral Guide

Remember when doctors laughed at vitamin pills? Not anymore. It's looking like supplements may help ward off everything from heart disease, colon cancer, and diabetes to Alzheimer's, pneumonia and colds, cataracts, osteoporosis, and more.

Fantastic! But how do you find the right products—and avoid risky or useless ones? With this guide, you'll see at a glance how much is enough and how much is too much of all the essential vitamins and minerals.

As always, make healthy food your mainstay—no pills can match it. But for smart nutrition insurance, the right supplements make sense, too.

What Is a Safe Upper Limit?

The figures in column three of the table are not your recommended goals—that's what the Daily Value (DV) is. But if you decide to exceed the DV, stay within the Safe Upper Limit. It represents the maximum intake unlikely to pose health risks, based on studies of people who have taken these amounts. Levels marked with ★ are new Tolerable Upper Intake Levels (ULs for short) set by the Food and Nutrition Board of the National Academy of Sciences. More are on the way. Other levels, unless noted, come from *Vitamin and Mineral Safety*, by John Hathcock, Ph.D., a respected

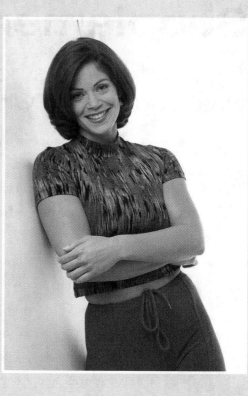

authority on vitamin and mineral toxicology. (*Vitamin and Mineral Safety* was issued in 1997 by the Council for Responsible Nutrition, a supplement industry group. It is posted on the council's Web site, at www.crnusa.org.)

"If there's no UL, *Vitamin and Mineral Safety* is a good guide," says John Erdman, Ph.D., director of the division of nutritional sciences at the University of Illinois at Urbana-Champaign.

Essential Vitamins and Minerals

Vitamin or Mineral	Daily Value (DV)/ Recommended Intake	Safe Upper Limit	What to Look for in a Multi	Good to Know
VITAMIN A Critical for healthy eyes and skin	5,000 IU	10,000 IU	Aim for 100% DV; all or part may be from beta-carotene	—
THIAMIN Helps your body turn carbohydrates into energy	1.5 mg	50 mg	Aim for 100% DV	High levels of thiamin, riboflavin, niacin, and B_6 are sometimes sold as "stress" formulas; there's no evidence that they help relieve stress
RIBOFLAVIN Helps produce energy in all of your cells	1.7 mg	200 mg	Aim for 100% DV	By law, white bread is enriched with riboflavin (as well as thiamin, niacin, iron, and folic acid)
NIACIN (NICOTINIC ACID) Helps your body use sugars and fatty acids	20 mg	35 mg*	Aim for 100% DV	Take higher levels only under a doctor's care
VITAMIN B_6 (PYRIDOXINE) Helps produce antibodies that fight infection	2 mg	100 mg*	Aim for 100% DV; most women's diets run short on B_6	Too much B_6 can cause reversible nerve damage
VITAMIN B_{12} (COBALAMIN) Helps make the protective lining of nerve cells	6 mcg	3,000 mcg	Aim for 100% DV, especially if you're age 50 or over	As you age, you absorb B_{12} better from supplements than from food
FOLIC ACID Critical for making DNA for new cells; helps reduce high blood levels of homocysteine	400 mcg	1,000 mcg*	Aim for 100% DV; it's unlikely that your diet provides enough; top sources are beans and other legumes, orange juice, and spinach	This is a must for women capable of bearing children; it's proven to cut nervous system birth defects in half; folic acid may also fight heart disease and colon cancer; excess folic acid from supplements can cause progressive neurologic damage in individuals with vitamin B_{12} deficiency
BIOTIN Helps your body turn food into energy	300 mcg	2,500 mcg	Ignore; your diet has enough†	Bacteria in your intestine also produce biotin
PANTOTHENIC ACID Helps your body turn food into energy	10 mg	1,000 mg	Ignore; your diet has enough†	Pantos means "everywhere" in Greek—and pantothenic acid is found in most foods

(continued)

Essential Vitamins and Minerals—Continued

Vitamin or Mineral	Daily Value (DV)/ Recommended Intake	Safe Upper Limit	What to Look for in a Multi	Good to Know
VITAMIN C Keeps your immune system, gums, and capillaries healthy	60 mg	1,000 mg	Aim for 100% DV; add C supplement of between 100 and 500 mg	Only humans, guinea pigs, and monkeys need to get vitamin C; other animals make their own; excess vitamin C may cause diarrhea in some people
VITAMIN D Makes it possible for you to absorb calcium from food	400 IU; people over 50 may need up to 800 IU	2,000 IU*	Aim for 100% DV; choose a calcium supplement with vitamin D	Research hints that vitamin D helps keep arthritis in check
VITAMIN E Neutralizes free radicals that can cause heart disease and cancer	30 IU	400 IU	Aim for 100% DV; add E supplement of between 100 and 400 IU	If you take blood-thinning medication or aspirin, consult your doctor before taking E; one small study showed a possible risk of hemorrhagic stroke in dosages higher than 200 IU, so consult your doctor if you are at high risk for stroke
VITAMIN K Essential for your blood to clot	80 mcg	30,000 mcg (30 mg)	Aim for 25 mcg; many multis unfortunately omit K	If you're on blood-thinning medication such as warfarin (Coumadin), tell your doctor before taking K
CALCIUM Essential for strong bones, and to fight high blood pressure, colon cancer, and PMS	1,000 mg (age 50 and over: 1,500 mg§)	2,500 mg*	Aim for 200 mg; no multi will have 100% DV; then add a calcium supplement (500 mg if you're 50 or under; 1,000 mg if you're over 50)	If you don't get enough dietary calcium, your body pulls it from your bones
COPPER Needed for healthy connective tissue in heart and blood vessels	2 mg	9 mg	Aim for 100% DV; most women's diets are very short on copper	Try to keep percent of DV of copper and zinc close to equal
CHROMIUM Works with insulin to help your body use blood sugar	120 mcg	200 mcg	Aim for 100% DV; few multis have this much, so you may need to settle for less	The only reason to take more than 200 mcg is if you have diabetes (to control blood glucose); be sure this is done under a doctor's care
IODINE Part of a thyroid hormone that regulates the rate of energy burn	150 mcg	1,000 mcg	Aim for 100% DV	Most dietary iodine comes from using iodized salt
IRON Part of hemoglobin, which carries oxygen to every cell in your body	18 mg	65 mg	Women with heavy periods, aim for 100% DV; men, all other women, look for no-iron or low-iron (0–9 mg) formula	Don't take iron above the DV unless a blood test says you're anemic; high iron intake may be linked to heart disease

Vitamin or Mineral	Daily Value (DV)/ Recommended Intake	Safe Upper Limit	What to Look for in a Multi	Good to Know
MAGNESIUM Needed for strong bones, and healthy nerves and muscles	400 mg	350 mg*	No multi has 100% DV, so aim for 100 mg; plus, eat lots of cooked dried beans, whole grains, and spinach	Don't take more than 350 mg from supplements; higher amounts can cause diarrhea in some people; people with heart or kidney problems should check with their doctors before taking supplemental magnesium
MANGANESE Part of many enzymes that control the chemical reactions in your body	2 mg	10 mg	Ignore; your diet has enough†	Whole grains are the best food sources
MOLYBDENUM Helps your body make hemoglobin	75 mcg	350 mcg	Ignore; your diet has enough†	Molybdenum deficiency has not been found in humans
PHOSPHORUS Part of your DNA and your genes; also part of your bones (second only to calcium)	1,000 mg	Age 70 and under: 4,000 mg;, over age 70: 3,000 mg*	Ignore; your diet has enough (including some from additives in processed food)	So prevalent in foods that deficiencies are extremely rare
POTASSIUM Helps maintain normal blood pressure	3,500 mg	3,500 mg‖	Multis contain tiny amounts; make sure you eat lots of vegetables and fruit	Because of potential serious risks, take potassium supplements only under a doctor's care
SELENIUM Protects cells from free radicals that can cause cancer and heart disease	70 mcg	200 mcg	Aim for 100% DV—but since many multis have less, you may need to settle for less	People taking 200 mcg a day cut their risk of lung, prostate, and colorectal cancer in half, one study found (May be toxic at 1,000 mcg)
ZINC Important for wound healing and a strong immune system	15 mg	30 mg	Aim for 100% DV; zinc is one of the minerals most lacking in U.S. diets	Too little zinc weakens immunity; but so does too much

*Tolerable Upper Intake Level (UL)

†It won't hurt you to get more from your multi, but there's no sign that American diets are deficient

‡Since no DV (set by the FDA) exists for this nutrient, this is the level recommended by the Food and Nutrition Board

§For adults age 50+, the National Institutes of Health recommends 1,500 mg daily

‖From personal communication with David A. McCarron, M.D., professor of medicine at Oregon Health Sciences University in Portland

Three Bright Stars

In addition to the basics, the latest research is emphasizing the health benefits of three more nutrients often in short supply in your diet and in good multivitamins. Consider taking the following minerals as separate supplements.

Caution: People with abnormal kidney function should check with their doctors before supplementing with minerals.

Magnesium. Single-dose multis don't go above 100 milligrams (mg) of this mineral. And the foods in which this is most abundant—whole grains, soybeans, and nuts, for example—aren't eaten with the regularity that would ensure adequate intake. But magnesium is important: The diseases it could protect you from are all killers: diabetes, heart disease, high blood pressure, and osteoporosis. It may also help relieve migraines. Aim for a total of 350 mg from both your multi and a supplement. (More than that may cause diarrhea.)

Chromium for diabetes. It's hard to get the Daily Value (DV) of 120 micrograms (mcg) of chromium from food alone. Even many multis come up short. But chromium is absolutely vital to helping your body process glucose for energy. Low levels of chromium may

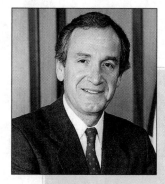

HEALING SPOTLIGHT
Senator Tom Harkin

Senator Tom Harkin, a Democrat from Iowa, was the driving force behind the creation of the Office of Alternative Medicine, which was established in 1992 under the auspices of the National Institutes of Health (NIH). Several personal experiences, among them his belief that bee pollen supplements cured his own severe allergy problems, convinced Harkin that alternative therapies have merit. He now watches his diet carefully and takes, in addition to the bee pollen, daily supplements of vitamins A, C, and E, plus saw palmetto for his prostate.

Senator Harkin says he is far from the only member of Congress who has made natural healing a part of his life. "There's much more receptivity on the Hill now than there used to be. It has to do with individual members who have used alternative therapies that worked, or whose spouses have. And I think Congress simply mirrors the American people. As more and more Americans are using alternative therapies, so are members of Congress. And that has added a great deal of weight to our efforts to have the NIH take alternative methods seriously."

increase your risk of type-2 diabetes, and studies suggest that 200 to 1,000 mcg of chromium can improve your symptoms if you have the disease. But more studies on long-term supplementation still need to be done. Don't go above 200 mcg without first checking with your doctor.

Selenium. This antioxidant is showing great promise as a cancer fighter. One 10-year study of 1,300 people found that those who took 200-mcg supplements cut their rate of overall cancer by 39 percent and their rates of lung, prostate, and colon cancers nearly in half. Don't exceed 200 mcg total, including the amount in your multivitamin.

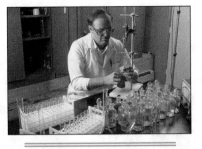

"Though scientific data and popular interest have increased, the amount of information that medical students receive about supplements—or indeed, the entire field of nutrition—is hardly greater now than it was 30 years ago when I was in school."

—James S. Gordon, M.D.,
Manifesto for a New Medicine

that the combination reduces pain and slows down cartilage loss in osteoarthritis, the wear-and-tear form of arthritis that causes aching, deteriorating joints. Alternative health practitioners and even some mainstream docs in the United States have also reported some success with the combo.

The word "cure" is an overstatement, though. In Hendersonville, North Carolina, orthopedic surgeon Amal Das, M.D., is analyzing data from a study he recently completed. "The combination was significantly effective for pain relief in people with mild to moderate arthritis," he says, "but not for severe arthritis."

Follow label directions for dosages. You can get the two supplements either separately or as a combination. But be careful what you buy: A University of Maryland study found a few products that contained far less glucosamine or chondroitin than the labels claimed. Two combination products that passed the study's quality tests were Cosamin DS and Joint Fuel. If you try them, tell your doctor. Give the supplements 8 weeks to work—it often takes that long. If you don't see any improvement by then, stop using them. So far, both glucosamine and chondroitin appear safe.

The Up-and-Comers

These nonnutrient supplements are the headline grabbers. While preliminary research looks good, they're not for everyone. Many health experts want to see more studies before recommending them.

Glucosamine and chondroitin. Your body makes these two substances to help build and protect cartilage, the shock-absorbing cushion that caps the ends of your bones. Preliminary studies, mostly European, have shown

Alpha-lipoic acid (ALA). A relative newcomer to the market, ALA is an antioxidant that your body normally makes on its own. It helps break down food into the energy needed by your cells. Supplementing may be helpful if you have or are at high risk for diabetes, because your energy metabolism is impaired. Preliminary studies suggest that ALA prevents the nerve damage in the lower legs that often occurs as the result of diabetes, possibly because of its protective effect on the smaller blood vessels.

The effective dosage in one recent study of people with diabetes was 800 mg a day for 4 months. No adverse effects were reported.

Coenzyme Q$_{10}$. CoQ$_{10}$ is another antioxidant manufactured by the body, where it goes by the name ubiquinone. This supplement claims many healing powers. Right now, however, CoQ$_{10}$'s potential benefits appear limited to helping you if you have or are at risk for congestive heart failure, which occurs when your heart is too weak to pump blood to your lungs and the rest of your body. It may also be good for gum disease, a leading cause of tooth loss.

One study found that 150 mg per day protected some people with congestive heart failure. (People using that amount were hospitalized 38 percent less than people on placebos.) And 50 to 60 mg a day helped reverse gum disease.

Caution: While CoQ$_{10}$ appears safe, congestive heart failure and gum disease (gingivitis) are not do-it-yourself diseases. They require a doctor's care.

Take a Pass

Some supplements remain mysteries yet to be solved by further research. And some, based on a lack of evidence so far, don't justify the expense.

Everyday Supplements

There's no escaping it: The best preventive medicine is a great diet and regular exercise. But many diets shortchange important nutrients, so it's also smart to take a multi supplement that contains 100 percent of the Daily Values (DV) for most essential vitamins and minerals. (No multi contains them all.) Take with meals for best absorption.

In Your Daily Multivitamin/Mineral Supplement

Vitamin A/beta-carotene (5,000 international units, or IU)
Vitamin B$_6$ (2 milligrams, or mg)
Vitamin D (400 IU)
Folic acid (400 micrograms, or mcg)
Magnesium (100 mg)
Zinc (15 mg)
Copper (2 mg)
Chromium (120 to 200 mcg)

Shark cartilage. While you can't write off this tabloid supplement yet, it's too soon to start taking shark pills to ward off cancer. Promoters speculate whether shark cartilage can prevent cancer by blocking blood vessel growth in tumors, depriving them of nutrients to grow. But there are no well-controlled studies to support this. And forming new blood vessels isn't al-

Selenium (at least 10 mcg; DV is 70, but most multis contain less) *Caution:* Unless you have iron-deficiency anemia, look for a multi with no iron. You probably don't need extra iron, and recent studies have linked high iron levels with increased risk of heart attack and atherosclerosis (a buildup of fatty deposits on your arteries).

In Addition

Plus, take these every day: You won't find the optimal dose of the following nutrients in any multi, so buy them separately.

Vitamin C (500 mg a day). You can get this from foods, but will you? Studies suggest that C supplements taken for 10 years reduce cataracts by more than 75 percent.

Vitamin E (100 to 400 IU). This is the only way to get the amount of E that may protect you from heart attacks, colds and flu, prostate and colon cancers, diabetes, and Alzheimer's disease. If you take blood-thinning medication or aspirin, consult your doctor before taking E. One small study showed a possible risk of hemorrhagic stroke in dosages higher than 200 IU. Consult with your doctor if you are at high risk for stroke.

Calcium (500 mg if you're age 50 or under; 1,000 mg if you're over age 50). Along with dietary calcium, this should bring you up to recommended levels to fight osteoporosis. Over age 50, look for a formula with vitamin D—you may need more D than your multi supplies.

Take calcium carbonate (the least expensive calcium) with meals; you can take calcium citrate on an empty stomach. For the best absorption, don't take more than 500 mg at one time.

ways a bad thing, points out Alan R. Gaby, M.D., professor of nutrition at Bastyr University in Seattle. It's useful when your cardiovascular system is trying to move blood around blockages, for example, or during pregnancy or for wound healing. Dr. Gaby also doubts that popular oral supplements of shark cartilage can even make it into the bloodstream, because their active ingredient is a protein that is destroyed by digestion.

Blue-green algae. This supplement comes in more than 1,000 different strains that grow in lakes and oceans. The algae available as a supplement generally began life in a lake as pond scum. They do contain protein, B vitamins, and minerals. But algae leave a lot of nutrition experts cold. You can get plenty of those same nutrients from food and a multi, notes Dr. Gaby. There have also been reports of toxicity, contamination, and illness associated with some algae.

Chromium for weight loss. Theoretically, it could work, says Priscilla Clarkson, Ph.D., professor of exercise science and associate dean of the University of Massachusetts School of Public Health in Amherst. "Chromium enhances insulin action. And insulin aids fat metabolism. That means chromium could potentially burn fat. But that theory hasn't yet become fact." Studies showing that supplemental chromium takes off the pounds have been weak or inconsistent.

Chelated supplements. Chelation is simply a technique for binding minerals with another substance that's supposed to enhance mineral absorption by the body. But actual studies proving better absorption are few. Specific use of the word "chelated" on a mineral supplement is often just a marketing buzzword to make you think it's better than the rest, says Dr. Gaby.

NATURAL HEALING THROUGH HISTORY

Linus Pauling: A Founding Father

By the time he was 61, Linus Pauling had won two Nobel prizes, one for his work in chemistry, the other for his work for peace. At that point, he was ready to get down to business, helping to launch the modern vitamin and supplement movement.

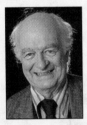 Pauling had theorized for much of his career about the possibilities of using relatively huge doses of vitamin C to treat colds and other diseases. In 1970, he published *Vitamin C and the Common Cold*, and the American sniffle would never be the same. The book, together with subsequent books that expanded his claims about the benefits of vitamin supplements to include cancer and heart disease, was enormously influential, and not just because it alerted the public to the possible health benefits of vitamins. Pauling also helped shift the focus of American health care away from the treatment of disease to its prevention. By emphasizing that it was important to support what he referred to as "the body's natural protective mechanism," he was one of the earliest advocates of what would evolve into today's natural-healing revolution.

Like most pioneers, Pauling encountered voracious opposition from the establishment. "Pauling's nutrition comments of recent times have disappointed us," wrote a doctor who worked for the Harvard School of Public Health, "not only because they make no sense in terms of modern medicine or nutrition but also in the irresponsible way they arouse false hopes in those who have diseases which Pauling feels can be successfully treated by his 'vitamin therapy.'" For nearly 30 years, Pauling and his critics traded research studies, each claiming to validate his own views for or against the efficacy of vitamin C. Definitive proof that it worked as Pauling said it did was hard to come by, but Pauling never backed down. "I am just too stubborn to change my mind about anything under pressure," he said.

Gradually, the tide shifted in Pauling's favor. Many scientists are now convinced that vitamin C and other antioxidants can be extremely important tools for fighting a host of diseases, including colds and cancer. Pauling enjoyed not only the last laugh but also the benefits of practicing what he preached. He died of prostate cancer at the age of 93, claiming that he would have died 20 years earlier if it hadn't been for vitamin C. Each day at breakfast, he stirred 12,000 milligrams into his orange juice. That's about 200 times the government's recommended Daily Value.

Chapter 8

Fight Disease with Teamwork

Put vitamins, minerals, and diet together to fight four major killers

Teamwork. It's the underlying principle that defines what natural health care in the twenty-first century is all about. We now have the luxury of bringing a broad range of tools and disciplines to bear on any given health issue. None of these elements needs to be pursued to the exclusion of the others. Balance and harmony are key.

Supplements and diet are a perfect example of how the new holistic medicine can be applied. Consuming a steady diet of junk food and trying to make up for it by gobbling down handfuls of vitamins won't cut it. To get the nutrients your body needs, a healthy diet is essential. But you can augment the benefits of that diet by taking supplements. That's why they call them supplements, after all.

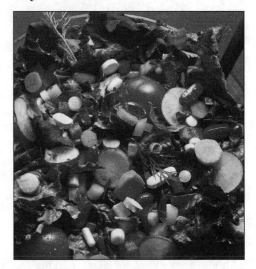

Now, let's take this teamwork principle a giant step further.

A Customized Plan

Many of us have a family history that suggests we may be at higher-than-average risk of developing one of the four diseases that kill more Americans than any others: heart disease, stroke, cancer, and diabetes. It makes sense, if you're at risk for one of those diseases, to employ all the tools at your disposal to stack the odds in your favor.

You can do that, simply and naturally, by customizing a diet-and-supplement regimen that will help your body fight the diseases that genetically threaten you. That's how holistic health care works. Here's how experts suggest turning an ordinary healthy diet into one that's literally death defying.

The first step in designing your own disease-fighting diet is to build a sound foundation. We recommend that you follow "*Prevention's* Basic Healthy Eating Plan," described on page 64. Once you have those fundamentals covered, you can begin to zero in on the high-risk disease that concerns you by following the specific regimens provided here.

If you're worried about all four diseases, don't panic. You don't need to eat 22 hours a day in order to get your nutrients. There's plenty of room in our basic eating plan to incorporate all the necessary foods into an optimal disease-fighting diet—without also increasing your waistline.

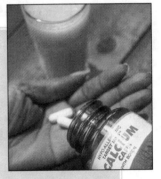

Safety with Supplements

Like prescription and over-the-counter drugs, any kind of supplement needs to be taken responsibly, says Mark Stengler, N.D., a naturopathic doctor and author of *The Natural Physician*. Before you start taking any supplements that are new to you, heed his following suggestions.

• To avoid or minimize any side effects, start with a lower dosage than the one stated on the label, then gradually increase the dosage until you reach recommended levels.

• Consult a knowledgeable physician or health practitioner before using any new supplements. Certain vitamins, herbs, and emerging dietary supplements can be toxic in higher doses.

• If you are pregnant or nursing, avoid all supplements unless they have been prescribed or approved by your doctor. Also, check with your physician before using supplements if you are taking prescription medication. People who are taking anticoagulant (blood-thinning) medications, for example, should not take high dosages of vitamin E, the herb red clover, and a number of other supplements that thin the blood.

Heart Disease and Stroke

To lower your risk, make sure you get these nutrients.

Folic acid (400 micrograms per day). Folic acid helps protect you by decreasing blood levels of the amino acid homocysteine, an emerging risk factor for heart disease and stroke, says Eric B. Rimm, Sc.D., assistant professor of epidemiology and nutrition at Harvard School of Public Health. Lots of foods contain folate (the folic acid naturally found in foods), including orange juice, kidney beans, broccoli, and spinach. But to make sure you get 400 micrograms (mcg), *Prevention* recommends taking a multivitamin that contains that amount.

Vitamin B$_6$ (3 milligrams per day). Like folic acid, vitamin B$_6$ helps reduce homocysteine levels. Taking supplements is probably a good idea because many people don't even manage to get enough to cover the 2 milligram (mg) Daily Value (DV), according to Walter Willet, M.D., Dr. P.H., chair of the department of nutrition at Harvard School of Public Health.

Foods containing B$_6$ include bananas, avocados, lean chicken, brown rice, and oats. The same multivitamin that provides your DV of folic acid can ensure that you get enough B$_6$.

Vitamin E (400 international units, or IU, per day). There's no shortage of studies showing that vitamin E in amounts ranging from 100 to 800 IU may reduce your risk of heart disease by about 40 percent. Doctors believe that the antioxidant properties of vitamin E stop the changes in your "bad" low-density

lipoprotein (LDL) cholesterol that make it more likely to clog your arteries. If you are considering taking this amount of vitamin E, discuss it with your doctor first. One study using low-dose supplements showed increased risk of hemorrhagic stroke.

To get the necessary amount of E, you probably need a supplement. The best sources of the heart vitamin are vegetable oils, nuts, and wheat germ, but you'd have to eat unhealthy quantities to even approach the amount recommended to prevent heart disease.

Prevention's Basic Healthy Eating Plan

These recommendations are the building blocks for a healthy, disease-fighting diet.

- Aim for 25 percent of calories from fat, 60 to 65 percent from carbohydrates, and 10 to 15 percent from protein.
- Eat a maximum of one serving (3 ounces) of lean meat, but preferably not every day. One cup of beans can count as a serving of meat.
- Minimize added fats, oils, foods with added sugar, and processed foods.
- Stay under 300 milligrams of cholesterol.
- Stay under 2,400 milligrams of sodium.
- Shoot for 20 to 35 grams of fiber.

Omega-3 fatty acids (3 ounces of salmon, mackerel, haddock, or another "fatty" fish once a week). That one meal could reduce your risk of cardiac arrest by 50 to 70 percent, according to the Journal of the American Medical Association. Fatty fish is packed with omega-3 fatty acids, substances that are believed to reduce heart spasms, and the clumping of blood platelets that leads to dangerous clots in your arteries.

From the Cutting Edge

Lycopene. A lot of people think of this as the spaghetti nutrient because it's so abundant in tomatoes and tomato products. In the last year or two, studies have shown that lycopene (one of a large family of carotenes of which beta is the most well-known) may help prevent heart disease and cancer. Just one or two servings a day will boost your lycopene levels into the high range. Cooked tomato products are higher in lycopene than raw, and it helps to consume a little fat, such as olive oil, to help your body absorb it.

Flavonoids. Think grapes. This fruit contains flavonoids shown to have blood-thinning abilities. One study found that drinking a 5-ounce glass of purple grape juice twice a day reduced the tendency for blood to clot by 60 percent. That was 50 percent better than the anticlotting ability of aspirin, considered the gold standard. If you're taking aspirin, however, it's still

NATURALFACT

Heart disease kills women five times more frequently than breast cancer does. Despite that, when it comes to screening for heart disease, doctors test women less frequently than men and recommend lifesaving heart surgery less often.

too soon to banish it to the medicine cabinet in favor of grape juice.

You may also want to eat more apples and onions, two other foods that contain high levels of flavonoids. Finnish researchers found that people who ate the greatest amounts of apples and onions had the lowest risk of heart disease. Tea also contains abundant flavonoids.

Cancer

To lower your risk, you need the following.

Fruits and vegetables. Five or more servings a day—but make them different foods of different colors. That's the best way to get all of the phytochemicals (phyto means "plant") associated with lower cancer risk.

Selenium. On average, men who took the mineral selenium in daily doses of 200 mcg for 4 years lowered their rates of lung, colorectal, and prostate cancer by more than half than men who didn't take it. Selenium's protective effects are probably due to its antioxidant properties. Don't exceed 200 mcg total, including the amount in your multi supplement. (Most multis contain less than 70 mcg.) Doses above this amount must be taken under medical supervision.

Carotenoids. These include beta-carotene and lycopene, found in many red, yellow, and orange fruits and veggies. Carotenoids have been linked to a decreased risk of many cancers, including prostate, lung, stomach, and endometrial cancers.

Less fat. Reduce to 20 percent or less.

Vitamin E (200 IU). Researchers at the Fred Hutchinson Cancer Research Center in Seattle found that men and women who took 200 IU of vitamin E per day had less than half the risk of getting colon cancer,

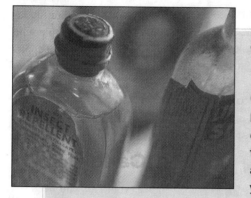

The Supplement Hall of Shame

Okay, we admit it. Supplements have had a rather checkered past. At one time or another, just about every-thing under the sun has been sold as a guaranteed remedy for what ails you. Here are some of the "healing" remedies that have been unloaded on an overly trusting public in years gone by. Definitely *don't* try these at home.

Swamp root. Made mostly of sugar and water colored with caramel, swamp root was touted to cure "acute and chronic diseases of the kid-neys, liver, bladder, urinary organs, and . . . all uric acid troubles."

Hadacol. Sold in the 1950s by Louisiana state senator Dudley J. LeBlanc, Hadacol's ingredients included a few vitamins, some honey, di-lute hydrochloric acid, and 12 percent alcohol. Supposedly, it cured anemia, arthritis, asthma, diabetes, epilepsy, gallstones, heart trouble, high blood pressure, low blood pressure, paralytic stroke, tuberculosis, and ulcers. It didn't.

The Hoxsey method. Harry Hoxsey inherited his secret cure for cancer from his father (who died of cancer, but we won't go into that). It consisted of an arsenic paste, which he would apply to the cancer area, where it would eat away the patient's flesh.

Kerosene. Kerosene was taken with a spoonful of sugar, mainly to treat colds, sore throat, and the croup. But some people claimed that it also cured pneumonia, convulsions, and diphtheria. They were probably mistaken.

compared to people who didn't take the vitamin.

Vitamin C. Diets high in vitamin C from fruits and veggies appear to protect against the risk of stomach, esophageal, mouth, and cervical cancers. We recommend adding 500 mg a day from a supplement, too.

From the Cutting Edge

Resveratrol. This substance found in ordinary grapes inhibits cancer growth by preventing three things: the start of DNA damage in a cell, the transformation of a normal cell into a cancerous one, and the growth and spread of tumor cells.

Although the study in which these findings appeared was done on laboratory mice, the results were so promising that the researchers believe this substance merits testing in humans as a potential cancer-preventing drug.

Catechins. These are the antioxidants found in tea, especially green tea. In animals, catechins inhibit a wide variety of tumors; ongoing human studies are now testing green tea against breast, prostate, and several other cancers.

Soy. Tofu and other soy-based foods contain high amounts of substances called isoflavones. At least in the test tube, researchers found that isoflavones could stunt the growth of human breast cancer cells by up to 30 percent.

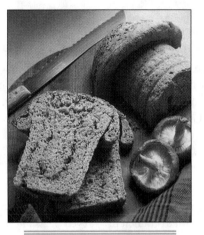

If you're at risk for diabetes, 60 percent of your diet should come from carbohydrates, including plenty of fruits, vegetables, beans, and whole grains.

Another study found that women who eat lots of soy products have less than half the risk of endometrial cancer of women who don't eat soy foods.

Diabetes (Type 2)

If you're at risk, you need the following.

Lots of fiber, little fat. Your diet should derive about 60 percent of calories from carbohydrates, preferably high-fiber, complex (unrefined) carbs such as fruits, vegetables, beans, and whole grains. You should also get no more than 25 percent of calories from fat, preferably unsaturated vegetable oils or monounsaturated olive oil, and 15 percent from protein.

High-fat diets increase your risk for obesity, the number one risk factor for diabetes. Refined carbohydrates that are rapidly absorbed, such as white bread, white rice, pasta, fruit juices, and soda, cause your blood sugar to shoot up, putting excessive stress on your pancreas to produce more insulin. By contrast, unrefined foods, which are high in fiber, are absorbed into your system more slowly, causing a gradual rise in blood sugar and a decreased need for insulin.

Chromium. This mineral helps make your cells receptive to insulin. Some studies show that it can help normalize glucose and insulin levels, too. Since it's hard to get the DV of 120 mcg of chromium from your diet, make sure you're getting 120 to 200 mcg from your daily multivitamin/mineral supplement. If you've been diagnosed with glucose intolerance, a condition that often leads to diabetes, USDA chromium expert Richard A. Anderson, Ph.D., recommends taking 200 mcg of chromium picolinate two or three times a day. Discuss with your physician first.

Magnesium. You need 350 mg total from your supplements. If your diet is deficient in magnesium (most are), you may be more resistant to insulin, putting you at risk for diabetes. People with heart or kidney problems should check with their doctors before taking supplemental magnesium. Supplemental magnesium may cause diarrhea in some people.

Harvard researchers found that the more magnesium in your diet, the less likely you are to get diabetes. Foods high in fiber are also high in magnesium. They include cereals, spinach, black-eyed peas, and beans.

NATURAL HEALING IN THE FUTURE

Beyond the Vitamin Pill

Judith S. Stern, Sc.D., R.D., professor of nutrition at the University of California at Davis, is past president of the American Society for Clinical Nutrition. Here, she discusses the changes she sees on the horizon for vitamin supplements.

Q: What have been the major trends in supplement research in the last several years?

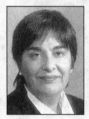

A: What has happened is that mainstream nutritionists now believe that we can't get it all from foods. That is, for optimal nutrition, some of us need to use supplements. For example, let's look at older women and calcium. Some of these women, especially those who don't eat many dairy products, find it tough to get the 1,000 to 1,500 milligrams of calcium that you need to keep osteoporosis risk minimal. As a result, we're seeing many nondairy foods, such as orange juice, supplemented with calcium. And we're also seeing many women resort to calcium supplementation.

Q: What's going on right now in the vitamin supplement field?

A: Antioxidants in general are very hot and will be for the foreseeable future, I can assure you. But what we're finding more and more with antioxidants is this: When we think we know what works and then put it in supplement form, it doesn't work. We find out it was something about the antioxidant in the food it was taken from that is the key to its healing power.

The classic example is beta-carotene. For awhile, we thought supplementation with beta-carotene could help protect us against cancer. Then one study conducted in Finland had an unexpected outcome. This study showed beta-carotene supplementation actually *increased* lung cancer risk. I used to take beta-carotene supplements myself. Not anymore.

Q: What's on the horizon?

A: At some point, I believe, we will get away from taking vitamin and mineral supplements and instead move toward eating formulated foods that already have in them the right amount of the vitamins and minerals that people need for specific health problems. The food manufacturers will offer formulated foods that are customized to different risk groups. So if you're a diabetic, you'll be able to choose from a menu of food offerings that have the right vitamin/mineral profile for diabetics.

This will be the revolution in vitamins, minerals, and antioxidants, I believe. We won't need to take them as supplements, which sometimes doesn't work anyway, as in the case of beta-carotene. Rather, we will get them in appropriate amounts in formulated foods that we can special order.

We always knew
that fresh fruits and
vegetables were good
for us. Now we're
finding out why.

Part Four

Miracle Foods

The same amazing powers that plants use to protect themselves can protect your health—and your family's.

Chapter 9

The Hidden Health Secrets of Plants

Unleash miraculous healing powers that can help your body fight disease

I t's not news that what we eat affects our health. What is news is that researchers are learning more each day just how powerful that food-health connection really is. Their discoveries are opening up a whole new understanding of how we can use food to prevent disease.

It turns out that in addition to vitamins and minerals, plants have a whole class of chemical properties called phytonutrients. These phytonutrients protect plants from their natural predators—insects, bacteria, viruses, and the like. Amazingly, when humans eat the plants that contain phytonutrients, they protect us, too. Not from bugs, but from things like high cholesterol, hardening of the arteries, heart disease, certain cancers, even aging itself.

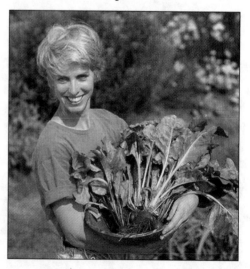

Blocking the Damage

The family of phytonutrients is a large one, and each member of this family works in different ways. Their most common weapons against disease, however, appear to be their antioxidant abilities.

Every day, your body is under attack by harmful substances known as free radicals. These are oxygen molecules that, due to pollution, sunlight, and everyday wear and tear, have each lost an electron. As they attempt to regain their missing electrons, they careen through your body, stealing electrons wherever they can. The molecular victims of these raids are damaged in the process and become free radicals themselves. Unless this chain reaction is stopped, the result is huge numbers of damaged molecules and, over time, irreparable damage and disease.

Here's an example. Normal cholesterol is a benign, helpful substance. But when cholesterol molecules are damaged by free radicals, they begin sticking to artery walls, causing hardened arteries and heart disease.

Another example: When free radicals attack molecules in your body's DNA, the genetic blueprint that tells your cells how to function, the blueprint is damaged. This is what allows cancer to develop. Even aging, many scientists believe, is caused by free radical damage.

The antioxidant powers of phytonutrients can quite literally save your life. Essentially, they step between the marauding free radicals and your body's cells, offering up their own electrons. When free radicals grab these "free" electrons, they become stable again and do no further damage. Most phytonutrients are potent antioxidants.

Who Said Life Was Fair?

It's called the French Paradox, and for years it has been one of science's greatest unsolved mysteries. Why is it that the French can continually indulge themselves in marvelous breads, rich buttery sauces, glass after glass of Burgundy, and all those unfiltered cigarettes and still have rates of heart disease that are 2½ times lower than ours? Now scientists think they know the answer: phytonutrients.

It seems that along with all the sinful stuff, the French are also consuming plenty of fresh fruits and vegetables, which are rich sources of a phytonutrient called flavonoids. Studies have shown that flavonoids can help stop the process that allows cholesterol to stick to artery walls, which is what eventually leads to blockages and to heart attacks.

To underscore the injustice of it all, flavonoids are also found in abundance in red wine.

Flushing Toxic Wastes

Another way that phytonutrients keep us healthy is by neutralizing and flushing toxic chemicals from our bodies before they have time to make us sick. They do this by manipulating enzymes known as phase-1 and phase-2 enzymes, explains Gary Stoner, Ph.D., director of the cancer chemoprevention program at the

The Miracle Nutrients

Why scientists always come up with such absurdly unintelligible names for things is one of life's great mysteries. The cataloging of the plant substances called phytonutrients is no exception. Still, they're names that you're bound to be hearing a lot more of, so we've made keeping track of them as easy as we can with the following chart. It lists some of the most important types of phytonutrients along with where you can find them and what they can do for you.

Phytochemical	Best Food Sources	Benefits
ALLYLIC SULFIDES	Onions, garlic	Raise beneficial HDL cholesterol; lower triglyceride (blood fat) levels; prevent heart disease; stimulate enzymes that suppress tumor growth
CAROTENOIDS	Carrots, broccoli, cantaloupe, greens, tomatoes	Act as antioxidants; prevent heart disease and certain cancers
FLAVONOIDS	Onions, kale, endive, citrus fruits, apples, broccoli, cranberries, red wine, grape juice	Act as antioxidants; prevent blood clots and heart disease
INDOLES and ISOTHIOCYANATES	Broccoli, cauliflower, cabbage, mustard greens	Stimulate cancer-preventing enzymes; block estrogen activity in cells
ISOFLAVONES	Soybeans, chickpeas, lentils, kidney beans	Block estrogen activity in cells; prevent certain cancers
LIGNANS	Flaxseed	Act as antioxidants; block estrogen activity in cells; may prevent certain cancers
MONOTERPENES	Citrus fruits, cherries	Prevent cancer by blocking certain cancer-causing compounds
PHENOLIC COMPOUNDS	Almost all fruits, vegetables, cereal grains, green and black teas	Act as antioxidants; activate cancer-fighting enzymes
SAPONINS	Soybeans, chickpeas, spinach, tomatoes, potatoes, nuts, oats	Bind with and flush out cholesterol; stimulate immunity; prevent heart disease and certain cancers

Ohio State University Comprehensive Cancer Center in Columbus.

Phase-1 enzymes are like double agents. They're created by your body and are important for normal cell function. But they have the ability to work against you, too. When cancer-causing toxins enter your system, phase-1 enzymes help make them active. Phase-2 enzymes, on the other hand, are real good guys. They seek out carcinogens and detoxify them before they do damage.

When you eat broccoli or other vegetables, some of the phytonutrients begin stomping out the enemy phase-1 enzymes while increasing the production of helper phase-2 enzymes. This process helps neutralize the various cancer-causing toxins that naturally accumulate in the body.

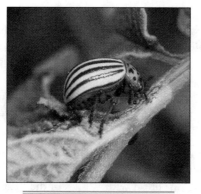

Phytonutrients protect plants from their natural predators—insects, bacteria, viruses, and the like. Amazingly, when humans eat the plants that contain phytonutrients, they protect us, too.

Hormone Helper

A third way in which some phytonutrients fend off disease is by keeping certain hormones—most notably, the female sex hormone estrogen—at healthy levels.

Estrogen also has a good side and a bad side. When it's produced at normal levels, it helps control everything from menstruation to childbirth. At the same time, it helps keep artery-clogging cholesterol in check, thus preventing heart disease. When estrogen levels rise, however, they can stimulate hormone-related cancers like those of the breast and ovaries, says Leon Bradlow, Ph.D., director of biochemical endocrinology at the Strang Cancer Research Laboratory in New York City.

There are several ways in which phytonutrients keep estrogen at its proper levels. For example, a class of phytonutrients called isoflavones are extremely similar to natural estrogen. When we eat foods containing isoflavones, they bind to the body's estrogen receptors, leaving the real hormone with nowhere to go but out.

Although estrogen is often referred to as if it were one hormone, there are, in fact, different forms. One kind of estrogen, called 16-alpha-hydroxyestrone, has been linked to breast cancer. Another form, 2-hydroxyestrone, appears to be harmless. Certain phytonutrients are able to increase levels of the harmless form of estrogen while decreasing levels of the dangerous kind, says Dr. Bradlow.

Eating Your Medicine

Add all these effects together, and it becomes clear that the disease-fighting powers of phytonutrients are staggering. As with vitamins and minerals before them, scientists foresee a day when many of these compounds will be used for treating disease in the hospital and for preventing it at home.

"People used to get beriberi, a vitamin-deficiency disease marked by a decline in neuro-muscular coordination, because they weren't getting enough thiamin in their diets," says Dr. Bradlow. "We started enriching our bread with thiamin, and now, nobody gets beriberi any-more. In the same way, it may be possible to develop high phytochemical–yielding strains of vegetables so that they can be used therapeuti-cally against diseases like cancer and heart disease."

In the meantime, researchers stress that there is only one way to get the phytonutrients that your body needs. You must eat them in the pack-ages Mother Nature provides: fruits, vegetables, and grains.

In the next chapter, we profile four of the richer sources of phytonutrients to spotlight how these miraculous substances work.

NATURAL HEALING THROUGH HISTORY

Beriberi: The Rice Mystery

It was a cruel experiment. In 1884, the director of the Japanese Naval Medical Bureau sent two ships on a 287-day voyage. The men on one ship ate meat, cooked fish, and vegetables, while the sailors on the other ship dined on the traditional Japanese diet of white rice and raw fish. All of the sailors on the first ship lived to see land, but almost half of the men on the other vessel came down with an illness called beriberi. Seventy-five died.

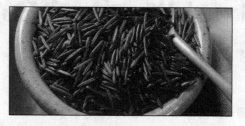

Beriberi causes terrible paralysis. The name *beriberi* translates to "I can't, I can't," which is how someone feels when he has it—that he really can't do anything. The disease had become common in the middle of the nineteenth century, but no one knew why. The theory at first was that some sort of virus had infected the food. Finally, researchers figured out that the problem wasn't what was in the food, but what *wasn't* in it.

The clue that solved the riddle came when someone noticed that two types of people seemed to be immune from the beriberi "virus": people who ate rice with the hull still intact and pregnant women who customarily ate boiled rice bran. Ordinarily, rice had its hull removed during the milling process. Now it was clear that something important was being lost with the hull. What, exactly, no one knew, but they knew enough to concoct a cure for beriberi by making a liquid extract of rice bran. They called it *tikitiki*.

The tikitiki cure helped establish that diet and disease were directly linked. In 1912, a Polish biochemist named Casimir Funk began studying the rice-beriberi connection. Eventually, he concluded that there was a single substance in our diets necessary for life, a substance he called "vitamines." The term was a combination of the Latin words for life ("vita"), and nitrogen ("amine"), since Funk believed that nitrogen was a component of this vital substance. Later research proved that there are not one, but many vitamins, and the final "e" was dropped in order to make the term more generic.

It was still a number of years before scientists would nail down specifically what the missing rice substance was that had led to the outbreaks of beriberi. It was thiamin, also known as vitamin B_1. (The name *thiamin* combines the Latin words for sulfur and nitrogen.) Today, we get thiamin in pork, ham, nuts, and whole-grain or enriched breads and cereals, and beriberi, at least in the West, is virtually nonexistent.

Chapter 10

Four Super Foods for Super Health

Powerful packages of vitamins, minerals, and phytonutrients—how they work

Phytonutrients. They don't sound that good, but they can taste good, very good. And they could save your life. Not a bad combination.

Although much remains to be learned about these phytonutrient compounds, a few are already showing tremendous promise. On the following pages, we profile four of the foods that scientists believe are among the richest of all sources of phytonutrients. These foods also happen to be chock-full of good old-fashioned vitamins and minerals. We call them Super Foods, and they're some of the best friends a body can have in fighting a host of diseases. We also provide you with some easy-to-prepare recipes that will help you get these Super Foods onto your table today, deliciously.

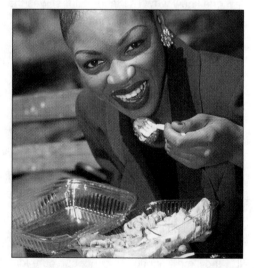

Beans: Small but Powerful

It wasn't so long ago that beans were second-class citizens on most American menus. Bags and cans of pinto beans, lima beans, chickpeas, black beans, kidney beans, and navy beans languished untouched on supermarket shelves, the same way three-bean salad sat untouched on picnic tables.

Not anymore. Americans' consumption of beans rose from 5.5 pounds per person in 1974 to 7.3 pounds in 1994. There's a good reason for this surge in popularity: Beans are the ultimate power food—low in fat and high in protein, fiber, and a variety of vitamins and minerals. Plus, they're packed with phytonutrients. All of that qualifies beans as one of the best health bargains you can buy.

Cancer-Licking Legumes

The phytonutrient punch packed by beans can inhibit the growth of cancer cells, studies suggest, by keeping normal cells from turning cancerous. Experts know that Hispanic women have about half the risk of getting breast cancer that Caucasian women face. Studies suggest that beans, which are eaten almost daily in many Hispanic households, may be responsible, says Leonard A. Cohen, Ph.D., head of the experimental breast cancer program at the American Health Foundation in Valhalla, New York. In one study, Dr. Cohen and his colleagues looked at the diets of 214 Caucasian, African-American, and Hispanic

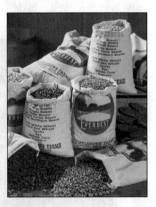

Beans: Shopping and Cooking Tips

Fiber favorites. While virtually all dried beans are good sources of fiber, some deliver more than others. Black beans, for example, contain 6 grams of fiber in a ½-cup serving. Chickpeas, kidney beans, and lima beans all weigh in at about 7 grams of fiber, and black-eyed peas are among the best, with about 8 grams of fiber.

Canned is fine. Don't have time to soak and cook dried beans? No problem. Canned beans are just as good for you as the dried kind. They're higher in sodium, however, so drain and rinse canned beans well before using them.

Defuse the gas. Don't let beans' unsavory reputation as gas generators stop you from enjoying their glories. Try spicing them with a pinch of summer savory or a teaspoon of ground ginger. According to some university studies, these spices may help reduce beans' gas-producing effects.

women. They found that the Hispanic women ate significantly more beans—7.4 servings per week, compared with 4.6 servings per week for the African-American women and less than 3 servings a week for the Caucasian women.

"Beans were a major source of fiber for the Hispanic women," says Dr. Cohen. In fact, the Hispanic women consumed nearly 25 percent of their dietary fiber from beans—twice the national average, noted the researchers.

Clear Out Cholesterol

To stay alive, we need to keep the coronary arteries, which supply life-giving blood to our hearts, clear of gunk. Cholesterol creates that gunk; beans can get rid of it. That's because beans are packed with soluble fiber, the same gummy stuff found in apples, barley, and oat bran. In the digestive tract, soluble fiber traps cholesterol-containing bile, removing it from the body before it's absorbed.

"Eating a cup of cooked beans a day can lower total cholesterol about 10 percent in 6 weeks," says Patti Bazel Geil, R.D., diabetes nutrition educator at the University of Kentucky in Lexington and author of *Magic Beans*. While 10 percent may not seem like much, keep in mind that every 1 percent reduction in total cholesterol means a 2 percent decrease in your risk for heart disease.

Beans can lower cholesterol in just about anyone, but the higher your cholesterol, the better they work. In a study at the University of Kentucky, 20 men with high cholesterol (over 260 milligrams per deciliter of blood) were given about ¾ cup of pinto and navy beans a day. The men's total cholesterol dropped an average of 19 percent in 3 weeks, possibly reducing their heart attack risk by almost 40 percent. Better yet,

Beans can help:

- Reduce the risk of breast and prostate cancers
- Lower cholesterol
- Stabilize blood sugar levels
- Prevent heart disease in people with diabetes

the dangerous low-density lipoprotein cholesterol—that's the artery-plugging stuff—plunged by 24 percent.

It appears that all beans can help lower cholesterol, even canned baked beans. In another University of Kentucky study, 24 men with high cholesterol ate 1 cup of beans in tomato sauce every day for 3 weeks. Their total cholesterol dropped 10.4 percent, and their triglycerides (another blood fat that contributes to heart disease) fell 10.8 percent.

Beans play another, less direct role in keeping cholesterol levels down. They're extremely filling, so when you eat beans, you'll have less appetite for other, fattier foods. And eating less fat is critical for keeping cholesterol levels low. "Beans are a high-fiber food, and high-fiber foods make you feel fuller," says Geil. In fact, one small study found that people who ate a bean puree felt more satisfied for a longer time than those who ate a similar puree made from potatoes.

Steady Your Sugar

Keeping blood sugar levels steady is the key to keeping diabetes under control. "Many people don't realize how good beans are for people with diabetes," says Geil. In fact, eating between ½ and ¾ cup of beans a day has been shown to significantly improve blood sugar control.

Beans are rich in complex carbohydrates. Unlike sugary foods, which dump sugar (glucose) into the bloodstream all at once, complex carbohydrates are digested more slowly. This means that glucose enters your bloodstream a little at a time, helping keep blood sugar levels steady, says Geil.

In addition, beans are high in soluble fiber. Studies have shown that a diet high in soluble fiber causes the body to produce more insulin receptor sites—tiny "docks" that insulin molecules latch on to. More insulin gets into individual cells where it's needed, and less is present in the bloodstream, where it can cause problems.

In an English study, people were given either about 1¾ ounces of a variety of beans—including butter beans, kidney beans, black-eyed peas, chickpeas, and lentils—or other high-carbohydrate foods, like bread, pasta, cereals, and grains. After 30 minutes, blood sugar levels in the bean eaters were almost half that of those who ate other high-carbohydrate foods.

The Healthy Meat

Beans used to be called the poor man's meat. But a more accurate name would be the healthy man's—and healthy woman's—meat. Like red meat, beans are loaded with protein. Unlike meat, they're light in fat, particularly dangerous, artery-clogging saturated fat.

For example, a cup of black beans contains

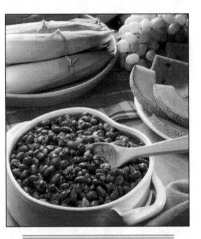

Eating a cup of cooked beans a day can lower total cholesterol about 10 percent in 6 weeks.

less than 1 gram of fat. Less than 1 percent of that comes from saturated fat. Three ounces of lean, broiled ground beef, on the other hand, has 15 grams of fat, 22 percent of which is the saturated kind.

Beans are also a great source of essential vitamins and minerals. A half-cup of black beans contains 128 micrograms, or 32 percent of the Daily Value (DV) for folate, a B vitamin that may lower risk of heart disease and fight birth defects. That same cup has 2 milligrams of iron, 11 percent of the DV, and 305 milligrams of potassium, or 9 percent of the DV. Potassium is a mineral that has been shown to help control blood pressure naturally.

Lentil Soup with Sun-Dried Tomatoes

This is a great immune-boosting recipe that is also easy to prepare—all the ingredients are probably right on your pantry shelf. If you're making this soup ahead, stir in the cooked pasta just before serving so that it won't absorb too much liquid.

1 Tbsp olive oil
1 large onion, chopped
2 garlic cloves, minced
4 cups reduced-fat, reduced-sodium chicken broth
3 cups water
2 cups dried lentils, rinsed

2 carrots, sliced
¼ tsp dried oregano
¼ tsp dried basil
¼ tsp dried rosemary
¼ tsp ground black pepper
½ cup oil-packed sun-dried tomatoes, drained and slivered
2 Tbsp balsamic vinegar
   Salt (optional)
1 cup very small shell pasta

Warm the oil in a soup pot over medium heat. Add the onion and garlic; sauté for 3 minutes. Add the broth, water, lentils, carrots, oregano, basil, rosemary, and pepper. Bring to a boil. Reduce the heat, cover, and simmer, stirring occasionally, for 20 minutes. Add the tomatoes. Simmer, stirring often, for 15 minutes, or until the lentils are tender. Stir in the vinegar. Season to taste with salt and more vinegar, if desired.

Meanwhile, cook the pasta according to package directions. Drain and stir into the soup.

Makes about 12 cups

Per 1½-cup serving: 312 calories, 18 g protein, 50 g carbohydrates, 7 g total fat, 1.5 g saturated fat, 0 mg cholesterol, 8 g fiber, 265 mg sodium

Black Bean Confetti Salad

This colorful and spicy salad looks as good as it tastes. Prepare it up to a day in advance if you like. Simply cover and refrigerate, then bring to room temperature before serving.

2 cans (15 ounces each) black beans, rinsed and drained
1 small red bell pepper, finely diced
4 scallions, thinly sliced
2 Tbsp fresh cilantro, chopped
2 Tbsp white wine vinegar
1 Tbsp extra-virgin olive oil

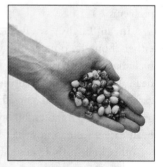

Too Busy for Beans?

A lot of people in this microwave era think they don't have time for all the soaking and boiling that dried beans require, but they haven't tried the quick-soak method. Here's how.

1. Rinse the beans in a colander, put them in a large pot, and cover with 2 inches of water. Bring to a boil, reduce the heat to medium, and boil for 10 minutes.

2. Drain the beans and cover with 2 inches of fresh water. (Discarding the water that the beans were cooked in gets rid of most of their gas-producing sugars, explains says Patti Bazel Geil, R.D., diabetes nutrition educator at the University of Kentucky in Lexington and author of *Magic Beans*.)

3. Soak for 30 minutes. Then rinse, drain, and cover with fresh water again. Simmer for 2 hours, or until the beans are tender.

In a large glass bowl, combine the beans, pepper, scallions, cilantro, vinegar, and oil. Let stand for 15 minutes to allow the flavors to blend.

Makes 4 main-dish servings

Per serving: 152 calories, 9 g protein, 26 g carbohydrates, 4.5 g total fat, 0.5 g saturated fat, 0 mg cholesterol, 8 g fiber, 589 mg sodium

Five-Star Vegetable Chili

This thick chili is loaded with phytonutrients, not to mention fiber, vitamin A, vitamin C, protein, and energy-giving complex carbohydrates.

- 1 tsp olive oil
- 1 onion, chopped
- 1 green bell pepper, chopped
- 2 garlic cloves, minced
- 1 jalapeño pepper, minced (wear plastic gloves when handling)
- 1 Tbsp dried oregano
- 2 tsp chili powder
- 1 tsp ground cumin
- 1 tsp ground coriander
- ¼ tsp ground red pepper
- 1 can (28 ounces) no-salt-added chopped tomatoes
- 1 can (15 ounces) no-salt-added tomato sauce
- 2 cups water

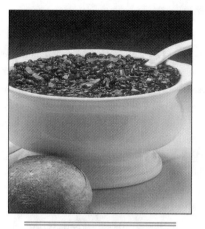

> **"Beans are actually little chemical factories with lots of biologically active substance in them, and there's good evidence that eating them may protect against cancer."**
>
> —Leonard A. Cohen, Ph.D., head of the experimental breast cancer program at the American Health Foundation in Valhalla, New York

- 2 tsp sugar
- ½ cup bulgur
- 1 can (14 ounces) cannellini beans, rinsed and drained
- 1 can (14 ounces) kidney beans, rinsed and drained

Warm the oil in a Dutch oven over medium heat. Add the onion and bell pepper. Cook, stirring occasionally, for 5 minutes, or until softened. Add the garlic and jalapeño pepper. Cook for 2 minutes, or until the vegetables are tender.

Warm a small no-stick skillet over medium-high heat. Add the oregano, chili powder, cumin, coriander, and red pepper. Stir for 1 to 2 minutes, or until fragrant. Add to the vegetable mixture. Add the tomatoes (with juice), tomato sauce, water, and sugar.

Increase the heat to medium-high and cook, stirring occasionally, for 5 minutes. Stir in the bulgur, cannellini beans, and kidney beans. Reduce the heat to medium and cook for 15 minutes, or until thickened.

Makes 4 servings

Per serving: 345 calories, 17 g protein, 67 g carbohydrates, 3 g total fat, 0.5 g saturated fat, 0 mg cholesterol, 16 g fiber, 574 mg sodium

Garlic: The Humble Bulb That Heals

You know garlic as the pungent spice whose odor you adore in Italian restaurants and detest on somebody's breath. What you might not be as aware of is the enormous amount of research documenting this humble bulb's status as one of the healing superstars of the plant world.

Studies show that garlic lowers cholesterol, thins the blood, kills bacteria, helps boost immunity, and reduces high levels of blood sugar. It may also relieve asthma and keep individual cells healthy and strong, perhaps delaying or preventing some of the conditions associated with aging.

It's fair to assume as well that the glorious taste of this humble bulb has powerful therapeutic effects on battered psyches, though hard data on that sort of thing is hard to come by.

A Growing Appreciation

Garlic's healing potential has been recognized for thousands of years, but only relatively recently has science come to appreciate the tremendous range of its powers.

Perhaps most impressive is garlic's double-action ability to help prevent heart attacks. First, it contains a type of phytonutrient called diallyl disulfide, or DADS. These are sulfur compounds that in the garlic plant act as a repellent to keep nibbling bugs away. In humans, they appear to keep blood flowing smoothly by preventing platelets from sticking together and clotting. Researchers at Brown University in Providence, Rhode Island, gave 45 men with high cholesterol aged garlic extract, about the equivalent of five to six cloves of fresh garlic. When they examined

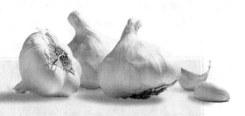

Garlic: Shopping and Cooking Tips

Enjoy it fresh. Crushed raw garlic contains allicin, a compound that breaks down quickly into a cascade of healthful compounds. Of course, not everyone enjoys the bite of raw garlic. Try cutting a clove in half and rubbing it hard against the inside of a wooden salad bowl before putting in the salad. You'll get just a hint of garlic taste and more than a hint of garlic benefits.

Eat for convenience. You don't have to prepare fresh garlic to get the healing benefits. Each form of garlic—raw, cooked, or powdered—has its own important compounds. By taking advantage of each of these forms, you can slip more garlic and its healing compounds into your menu.

Cut it fine. Whether you're cooking garlic or eating it raw, mincing, crushing, or pressing it vastly expands the surface area, maximizing the production and release of healthful compounds.

the men's blood, they saw that the rate at which platelets clumped and stuck together had dropped anywhere from 10 to 58 percent.

Garlic is also good for the heart because it lowers the levels of cholesterol and blood fats called triglycerides in the bloodstream. According to Yu-Yan Yeh, Ph.D., professor of nutrition science at Pennsylvania State University in University Park, many of garlic's protective effects take place in the liver, where cholesterol is produced. "The liver is a primary place in the body for fat synthesis and for production of blood cholesterol," says Dr. Yeh. "When fewer of these substances are made in the liver, there are fewer of them in the blood."

In a review of 16 studies involving 952 people, British researchers found that eating garlic—whether fresh or in powdered form—lowered total cholesterol an average of 12 to 13 percent.

Garlic against Cancer

A growing body of evidence suggests that garlic helps prevent the sorts of cell changes that can lead to cancer. Some of the phytonutrients in garlic appear to throttle the growth of cancer cells by interfering with their ability to divide and multiply. One compound is as effective at killing lung cancer cells as a widely used form of chemotherapy, opening the possibility that one day, garlic could form the basis of a new, gentler kind of cancer treatment.

These benefits are not just theories coming

NATURALFACT

In one study, researchers at Boston City Hospital swabbed 14 different strains of bacteria from the noses and throats of children with ear infections. Some of the infections had been impervious to treatment with antibiotics. In the laboratory, however, garlic extract effectively killed the resistant germs.

out of test tubes. Researchers have noted that people in southern Italy, who eat a lot of garlic, develop less stomach cancer than their neighbors to the north, who aren't as fond of garlic. Similar evidence has been noted closer to home. A study of 41,837 women living in Iowa found that those who ate garlic at least once a week had a 35 percent lower risk of colon cancer than women who never ate garlic.

"If I had to take an educated guess, I'd say that eating three cloves of garlic a day might reduce your risk of many cancers by 20 percent," says researcher Robert I. Lin, Ph.D., executive vice president of Nutrition International in Irvine, California. "And eating six cloves could get you at least a 30 percent reduction," he adds.

A Blessing for Ears

A frightening trend in recent years has been antibiotic resistance—the ability of bacteria to shrug off the effects of once-effective drugs. Recent research suggests that garlic may be effective where traditional drugs have failed or are too toxic.

In one study, researchers at Boston City Hospital swabbed 14 different strains of bacteria from the noses and throats of children with ear infections. Some of the infections had been impervious to treatment with antibiotics. In the laboratory, however, garlic extract effectively killed the resistant germs.

In another study, researchers at the University of New Mexico, Albuquerque, tested whether garlic could be used to treat otomycosis, or swimmer's ear. Swimmer's ear is caused, scientists think, by a fungus called *Aspergillus*. And normal treatments for it are less than ideal. Topical drugs can be uncomfortable and cannot be used if the eardrum has already been broken. In the laboratory study, researchers treated swimmer's ear fungi with a mixture of garlic extract and water. Even at very low concentrations, the garlic blocked the growth of fungi just as well as available drugs. And in some cases, it proved even better.

Garlic can help:

- Reduce the risk of stomach and colon cancers
- Prevent heart disease and stroke
- Lower cholesterol
- Ease ear infections

Mashed White Beans with Roasted Garlic

This is an interesting alternative to mashed potatoes. For the best result, use a bean that has a soft, creamy consistency, such as great Northern or cannellini.

    2   medium garlic bulbs
    2   Tbsp extra-virgin olive oil
    ¼   tsp salt
    ¼   tsp ground black pepper
    3   cups cooked white beans, cooking liquid
        reserved
    2   tsp finely chopped parsley
    2   tsp finely chopped fresh mint
    2   tsp finely chopped fresh basil
    ¼   cup grated Parmesan or Asiago cheese

Cut off the top quarter of the garlic bulbs to expose each clove. Drizzle them with 1 tablespoon of the oil and the salt and pepper. Wrap them in foil and roast in a 375°F oven for 30 minutes, or until the garlic is completely soft. (Uncover the bulbs for the last 5 minutes of cooking to allow the garlic to brown and caramelize.) Set aside.

In a food processor or blender, puree the beans, adding the reserved cooking liquid until the mixture resembles mashed potatoes. (The beans should not be completely smooth.) Heat the remaining 1 tablespoon oil in a skillet. Squeeze the roasted garlic out of its skin and into the skillet. Sauté the garlic briefly, then add the beans to warm them. Stir in the parsley, mint, and basil. Season with additional salt and pepper, if desired. Lightly top with the cheese.

Makes 4 side-dish servings

Per serving: 269 calories, 15 g protein, 34 g carbohydrates, 9.5 g fat, 2.5 g saturated fat, 5 mg cholesterol, 7 g dietary fiber, 259 mg sodium

Garlic Bean Spread

Roasting tempers and mellows garlic's heady flavor in this superb spread that may remind you of hummus. Serve with crackers or vegetable sticks.

    1   garlic bulb
    2   sun-dried tomato halves
    1   can (15½ oz) white beans, rinsed and drained
    1   tsp snipped fresh rosemary
    ⅛   tsp white pepper

Remove the papery skin from the garlic and coat the bulb with nonstick spray. Place in a small pan and roast in a 350°F oven for 30 to 40 minutes, or until soft and golden brown.

Meanwhile, soak the tomatoes in hot water for 10 minutes, or until soft. Drain, reserving 1 tablespoon of the soaking liquid. Chop the tomatoes.

Cool the garlic slightly and remove the cloves from their skins. In a food processor, process the garlic, tomatoes, reserved soaking liquid, beans, rosemary, and pepper until smooth. Cover and store in the refrigerator.

Makes 1½ cups

Per 2 Tbsp: 43 calories, 3 g protein, 9 g carbohydrates, 0.2 g fat, 0.5 g saturated fat, 0 mg cholesterol, 2 g dietary fiber, 93 mg sodium

Roasted Garlic and Vegetable Soup with Pasta

Adding lots of veggies to the garlic makes this soup one of the best friends your immunity system could have.

- 1 garlic bulb, separated and peeled
- 1 Tbsp olive oil
- 1 onion, diced
- 1 red bell pepper, diced
- 4 cups reduced-fat, reduced-sodium chicken broth

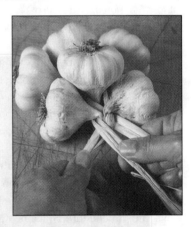

A Healthy Roast

Unless you have taste buds made of asbestos, it's difficult to eat a lot of raw garlic at one sitting. But there is a way to substantially boost your garlic intake without torturing yourself in the process. It's called roasting.

Unlike eating raw garlic cloves, roasting gives the bulb a sweet, caramelized taste—garlic at its most polite. It delivers just a hint of heat rather than the full blast.

To roast garlic, cut the top from the garlic bulb to expose just the tips of the cloves. Rub the bulb lightly with a little olive oil and wrap in a piece of aluminum foil. Leave some air space around the bulb, but seal the edges tightly. Roast in a 350°F oven for 45 minutes, or until very tender. (You can also "roast" garlic in the microwave oven. Microwave, uncovered and without oil, on high power for 10 minutes, turning twice during the cooking process.) Remove from the oven and let cool slightly.

To eat roasted garlic, simply squeeze the root end firmly to push the cloves out of their skins. You can spread the garlic on bread or toss it with cooked pasta or vegetables. If you're not eating it right away, you can refrigerate it in a tightly covered container for up to a week.

2 cups water
2 carrots, peeled and thinly sliced
1 Tbsp tomato paste
1 tsp dried basil
¼ tsp black pepper
4 cups shredded escarole
1½ cups tiny broccoli florets
1 cup elbow macaroni
¼ tsp salt (optional)
⅓ cup grated Parmesan cheese (optional)

Preheat the oven to 400°F. Allow the garlic to sit for 15 minutes. Wrap the garlic in foil and place in a small baking dish. Bake for 45 to 50 minutes, or until soft.

Warm the oil in a soup pot over medium heat. Add the onion and bell pepper. Sauté for 5 minutes. Add the broth, water, carrots, tomato paste, basil, and black pepper. Bring to a boil. Reduce the heat, cover, and simmer for 10 minutes.

Remove 1 cup of liquid. Mash the garlic into the liquid. Stir into the pot. Add the escarole and simmer for 7 minutes. Add the broccoli. Cover the pot and turn off the heat.

Cook the macaroni according to package directions. Drain and stir into the soup. If desired, season with the salt and sprinkle with the Parmesan.

Makes about 9 cups (6 servings)

Per 1½-cup serving: 148 calories, 7 g protein, 25 g carbohydrates, 3 g fat, 0.5 g saturated fat, 0 mg cholesterol, 4 g dietary fiber, 374 mg sodium

Discover the Phenomenal Joys of Soy

What if we told you that milkshakes will lower cholesterol, burgers can prevent cancer, and cheesecake will ease some of the bothersome symptoms of menopause?

Right, you'd probably answer. And where's the oceanfront property in Arizona you want me to look at?

Well, the fact is that all those healthy delights are possible, if you're using the humble soybean to make them.

Americans aren't very familiar with soy, but

The Breast Cancer Debate

You may have read about concerns that the weak estrogens in soy might actually stimulate breast cancer rather than fight it.

What's the truth? Seven experts in breast cancer and soy that *Prevention* contacted think that this is highly unlikely, though it is still being investigated. They point to many studies—in Asia, Australia, and the United States—that link diets high in soy with lower rates of breast cancer. None has ever linked a high-soy diet with more breast cancer.

As a sensible course, however, some experts advise women to stick with no more than one serving of soy a day until we learn more.

that will almost certainly change as word of this remarkable food's healing powers spreads. In Japan, where soy foods such as tofu and miso soup are dietary staples, deaths from breast cancer and prostate cancer are a fraction of what they are in the United States. And that's just the beginning of the joys of soy.

Good for Your Heart

Technically, we could have included soy in the section on beans, but soy is distinctive enough to stand on its own.

Its healing powers are extraordinary. Take, for example, soy's effectiveness as a cholesterol fighter. Japanese men have the world's lowest rate of death from heart disease, with Japanese women coming in a close second. A possible reason is that the Japanese eat about 24 pounds of soy foods per person per year. Americans eat an average of 4 pounds per person per year.

The association between tofu and lower cholesterol levels was affirmed by a meta-analysis, which complied and compared the results of 38 separate studies. The conclusion was that consuming 1 to 1½ ounces of soy protein (rather than animal protein) a day lowered total cholesterol by 9 percent and harmful low-density lipoprotein (LDL) cholesterol by 13 percent.

Menopause Medicine

More than half of American women in menopause complain of hot flashes and night sweats. In Japan, there isn't even a phrase for "hot flash." Might Japanese women have fewer

NATURALFACT

Not all soy foods contain the phytoestrogens that can help prevent breast cancer and osteoporosis. You won't find them in soy sauce or soybean oil, for example.

menopausal problems because they eat more soy?

Preliminary research suggests that's the case. In one study, researchers at the Brighton Medical Clinic in Victoria, Australia, gave 58 postmenopausal women about 1½ ounces of soy flour or wheat flour every day. After 3 months, the women eating soy flour saw their hot flashes plummet by 40 percent. Women given wheat flour, by contrast, had only a 25 percent reduction.

"If these data are confirmed," says Mark Messina, Ph.D., former head of the National Cancer Institute's Designer Foods Program, "then within a couple of years, we may be at a point where doctors say, 'Take 2 cups of soy milk per day' instead of recommending hormone-replacement therapy to relieve menopause symptoms."

Chest Protector

Researchers believe that the phytoestrogens in soy, which mimic a woman's natural estrogen, may help reduce the effects of the hormone in the body. Since estrogen is thought to fuel the growth of breast tumors, lower activity in the body could mean a lower risk of developing breast cancer.

The estrogens in soy can help protect women in several ways, depending on the stage of life. In premenopausal women, for example, a diet high in soy foods may lengthen the menstrual cycle. This is important, since every woman experiences a surge in estrogen at the beginning of her cycle. Multiplied over a lifetime, these surges expose the body to large amounts of estrogen, which eventually could cause cellular changes that lead to cancer. Lengthening the menstrual cycle, experts say, reduces the frequency of these surges, and with it, a woman's lifetime exposure to the hormone.

In one study, researchers at the National University of Singapore found that premenopausal women who consumed high amounts of soy foods, along with generous amounts of beta-carotene and polyunsaturated fats, had half the risk of developing breast cancer as women who consumed a lot of animal protein. Curiously, in women who are postmenopausal, soy foods appear to provide an estrogen "lift" that helps make up for the body's low levels of the hormone. This lift appears to provide the protective benefits of estrogen (such as helping to prevent osteoporosis) without raising the cancer risk.

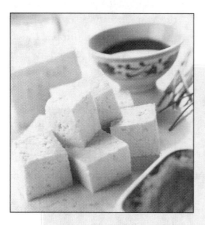

Soy: Shopping and Cooking Tips

Add it last. When cooking with tofu or other soy products, always add them late in the cooking process. Researchers speculate that cooking at high heats for extended periods of time may reduce or eliminate many of the nutritional benefits.

Shop for power. While it's best to eat soy foods in their unadulterated forms, there are times that you may have a taste for a ready-made vegetable burger or breakfast sausage. When buying processed soy foods, make sure that they contain "soy protein," "hydrolyzed vegetable protein," or "textured vegetable protein," which are all acceptable sources of protective plant compounds called phytoestrogens.

By contrast, don't expect too much from products containing soy protein concentrates, says James W. Anderson, M.D., professor of medicine and clinical nutrition at the Veterans Administration Medical Center at the University of Kentucky College of Medicine in Lexington. "Unfortunately, most of the beneficial substances are extracted from these products," he says.

Look for full-fat. While it's usually a good idea to reduce the amount of fat in your diet, full-fat soy milk contains 50 percent more phytoestrogens than the low-fat kind, says Dr. Anderson. "Getting those extra phytoestrogens is a good trade-off for the extra fat," he says.

Men's Problems

While most research exploring the protective effects of soy foods has looked at women, experts agree that men can benefit as well. It appears that soy reduces the harmful effects of the male hormone, testosterone, which is thought to fuel the growth of cancerous cells in the prostate gland.

A study of 8,000 Japanese men living in Hawaii found that those who ate the most tofu had the lowest rates of prostate cancer. Even though Japanese men develop prostate cancer just as often as Western men do, they nonetheless have the lowest death rates from prostate cancer in the world. Experts suspect that soy foods, by inhibiting the effects of testosterone, help shut off the "fuel" that causes cancers to grow.

The amount of soy that you need to enjoy these benefits appears to be tiny—one serving a day, according to Dr. Messina. "If that's for real," he says, "then soy could have a tremendous public health impact."

Nutritional Extras

It's easy to sound like a late-night TV salesman when it comes to the benefits of soy. "Wait! There's more!" It's true, though: In addition to all the phytonutrient protection that they provide, soy foods are just plain good for you from a nutritional standpoint.

For example, a half-cup of tofu provides about 20 grams of protein, 40 percent of the Daily Value (DV). The same half-cup supplies about 258 milligrams of calcium, more than 25 percent of the DV, and 13 milligrams of iron, 87 percent of the Recommended Dietary Allowance (RDA) for women and 130 percent of the RDA for men.

While soy foods are moderately high in fat,

Sinfully Soy

Here are four super-easy treats you can make yourself that will sneak soy deliciously into your diet.

Velvet latte. Heat 1 cup of plain or vanilla soy milk in the microwave oven for 1 minute, stir in a teaspoon of instant coffee, and soy milk becomes a smooth latte. Vanilla soy milk is sweet, so you won't need sugar.

Rich mocha latte. Use the same directions as above. But use 1 cup of chocolate soy milk. (We recommend White Wave Chocolate Silk.) This could become your favorite brew.

Extra-comforting cocoa. Make instant hot cocoa with 1 cup plain soy milk. What could be easier?

Heavenly chocolate-almond pudding. Use Mori-Nu Mates Chocolate Pudding/Pie Mix. Prepare according to the package directions with firm or extra-firm silken light tofu, but add ½ to 1 teaspoon almond extract. Bliss.

most of the fat is polyunsaturated. Soy foods contain little of the artery-clogging saturated fat found in meat and many dairy foods, says Dr. Messina.

Tofu and Brown Rice Casserole

This casserole's main ingredients may sound like something from a hippie commune, but there's nothing countercultural about the taste!

     2 Tbsp olive oil
     1 large onion, thinly sliced
     1 red bell pepper, thinly sliced
     1 green bell pepper, thinly sliced
     1 cup cooked brown rice
     1 tsp Italian seasoning
    12 ounces extra-firm tofu, drained and cut
        into cubes
        Dash of pepper
     1 cup fat-free milk
    ¼ to ½   cup whole-wheat bread crumbs
     2 ounces Parmesan cheese, grated

   Preheat the oven to 350°F. Heat the oil in a large skillet or wok over medium-high heat. Add the onion and bell peppers and cook for 5 minutes, or until lightly browned. Add the rice and Italian seasoning. Cook, stirring, for 2 minutes. Add the tofu and cook, stirring often, for 2 minutes. Place tofu mixture in a 1½- to 2-quart casserole coated with no-stick spray. Pour in the milk. Sprinkle with the bread crumbs or wheat germ and the cheese. Bake for 15 to 20 minutes, or until cheese is nicely browned.

   Makes 4 servings

   Per serving: 365 calories, 24 g protein, 27 g carbohydrates, 19.5 g total fat, 5 g saturated fat, 12 mg cholesterol, 5 g fiber, 5 mg sodium

Soy can help:

• Prevent heart disease
• Relieve menopausal symptoms
• Reduce the risk of breast cancer
• Ward off osteoporosis
• Prevent prostate cancer

Carrots Parmesan with Tofu

This makes a nice main dish for a light meal. Serve with a green vegetable or a green salad and fresh whole-wheat rolls and butter.

     1 cup mashed soft tofu
     ¼ cup fat-free milk
     1 egg
     ¼ cup Parmesan cheese
     ⅛ tsp pepper
        Dash of nutmeg
     5 large carrots, sliced and cooked until tender
     1 small onion, sliced very thin
     ½ cup cashews, chopped

   Preheat the oven to 350°F. Place the tofu, milk, egg, Parmesan, pepper and nutmeg in a food processor or blender. Pulse until smooth. Arrange the carrots and onion in a 1½-quart casserole coated with no-stick spray. Pour the tofu mixture over the carrots. Top with the cashews. Bake for about 30 to 35 minutes.

   Makes 6 servings

   Per serving: 195 calories, 12 g protein, 14 g carbohydrates, 11.5 g total fat, 3 g saturated fat, 39 mg cholesterol, 4 g fiber, 122 mg sodium

Charlotte's Chocolate Pudding

This delicious pudding is the creation of *Prevention* reader Charlotte Knipper of Dyersville,

Iowa. It makes a favorite dessert dish healthier, thanks to tofu. Blend it for a creamy style; use an electric mixer for more texture.

1 package (12.3 ounces) light silken tofu
1 package (1.4 ounces) instant sugar-free chocolate pudding mix
⅔ cup nonfat dry milk
1 cup prepared coffee, cold
1 tsp coconut extract (optional)
1 cup frozen fat-free whipped topping, thawed

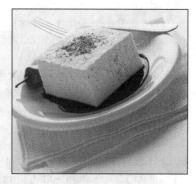

Six Ways to Enjoy Soy

Don't know tofu from tempeh? Here are some of the most common soy foods, along with a few suggestions for using them.

Meat substitutes. If you want to cut back on meat while getting more soy, look for "mock" meats, like cold cuts, bacon, sausage, franks, and burgers. These are mainly made from soy, and in some cases, they are virtually indistinguishable from the real thing.

Soy flour. Made from roasted ground soybeans, soy flour can be used to replace some of the wheat flour used for baking. Nutritionists advise buying defatted soy flour, which contains less fat and more protein than the full-fat variety.

Soy milk. A creamy, milklike drink made from ground soaked soybeans and water, it's sold plain and in a variety of flavors. Some people prefer "lite" soy milk. It's lower in fat than the regular kind, but it contains far fewer phytoestrogens.

Tempeh. These chunky, tender cakes are made from fermented soybeans that have been laced with mold, giving them their distinctively smoky, nutty flavor. You can grill tempeh or add it to spaghetti sauce, chili, or casseroles.

Texturized soy protein. Made from soy flour, this meat substitute can replace part or all of the meat in meat loaf, burgers, and chili.

Tofu. A creamy, white, soft cheeselike food made from curdled soy milk, tofu comes in firm and soft varieties and can be used in virtually anything from soups to desserts. You will find soft and firm tofu at most supermarkets in the produce section. Other soy foods are available at specialty and health food stores.

1 Tbsp finely chopped pecans
(optional)

Place the tofu in a blender and process until smooth. Add the pudding mix, milk powder, coffee, and coconut extract, if desired. Blend until smooth, scraping down the sides of the container as necessary. Transfer to a bowl. Fold in ¾ cup of the whipped topping.

Divide among 6 dishes. Chill for 30 minutes. Garnish with the pecans, if desired, and the remaining ¼ cup whipped topping.

Makes 3 cups

Per ½-cup serving:

90 calories, 7 g protein, 14 g carbohydrates, 1 g total fat, 0.04 g saturated fat, 1 mg cholesterol, 0 g fiber, 157 mg sodium

For Your Health's Sake, Go Green

What are greens? They're all the things that you didn't want to eat when you were a kid, and your mother insisted you had to because they were good for you. We're talking spinach, chard, and kale, mainly, plus dandelion greens, beet greens, mustard greens, turnip greens, and chicory greens.

Your mother was right, of course: greens are good for you, but nobody, including your mother, realized how good until recently. We now know that greens constitute a veritable tour de force of healthy vitamins, minerals, and phytonutrients. "These are the most nutrient-dense foods that we have available," says Michael Liebman, Ph.D., professor of human nutrition at the University of Wyoming in Laramie.

Greens can help:

- Control blood pressure
- Reduce the risk of heart disease
- Reduce the risk of cancer
- Protect against vision loss

Rabbit Heart

To some extent, the difference between people who have heart attacks and those who don't may be how many trips they make to the salad bar.

Researchers for one landmark study observed more than 1,000 people between the ages of 67 and 95 to learn what dietary factors affect heart health. They zeroed in on an amino acid called homocysteine which, when levels get too high, can become toxic, contributing to clogged arteries and heart disease. Guess what helped avoid that problem? You got it: leafy greens. It turns out that greens are excellent sources of two nutrients that help keep levels of homocysteine down: folate and vitamin B_6.

Boiled spinach is probably your best bet for managing homocysteine. A half-cup of Popeye's favorite snack delivers the 131 micrograms of folate, 33 percent of the Daily Value (DV). It also contains 0.2 milligram of vitamin B_6, 10 percent of the DV.

In addition to these important B vitamins, certain greens—particularly beet greens, chicory, and spinach—provide the heart-healthy minerals magnesium, potassium, and calcium. These minerals, along with sodium, help regulate the amount of fluid that your body retains. All too often, researchers say, people have too much sodium and too little of the other three, leading to high blood pressure.

Even though eating leafy greens is an excellent way to help regulate blood pressure, it's important to note that the calcium from spinach and beet greens isn't well-absorbed by the body. Be sure to eat a wide variety of greens to meet all your mineral needs.

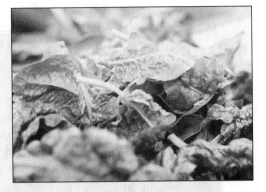

Greens: Cooking Tips

Many people wonder, should I cook my greens for flavor or not cook them to preserve their nutrients? It's a trade-off, says Michael Liebman, Ph.D., professor of human nutrition at the University of Wyoming in Laramie. "While it's great to eat them raw, you're more likely to eat more of certain vegetables if they're cooked. Just watch your cooking method. You don't want to boil them to death. Any quick-cooking method, such as blanching, is fine. One of the best cooking methods for retaining nutrients seems to be the microwave," he says.

Here are a few tricks for cooking greens successfully:

Trim the stems. While the leaves are often surprisingly tender, the stems on leafy greens can be unpleasantly tough and should often be discarded. Before cooking greens, run a sharp knife alongside the stem and center rib, separating the leaf from the stem.

Clean them well. Since the leafy greens grow close to the ground and the frilly leaves readily capture dirt and grit, it's important to wash them thoroughly. The easiest way is to fill the sink or a large bowl with cold water and swish the greens around, allowing any dirt or sand to sink to the bottom. When the greens are clean, transfer them to a colander to drain.

Cut them to ribbons. When cooking thick greens like kale or Swiss chard, it's helpful to cut them into ribbons or small pieces. This will help them cook quickly and become tender.

Boil them quickly. The easiest way to prepare greens is to submerge them in boiling water. Start with a cup of boiling water, drop in the greens, cover, and cook for 4 minutes, or until tender.

Cancer Fighter

The evidence is overwhelming that many types of cancer occur less frequently in countries where greens are a dietary staple and meat a rarity.

In one study, researchers compared 61 men with lung cancer with 61 men of similar age and smoking habits who were cancer-free. The one difference they found was that men with cancer consumed significantly fewer foods rich in a type of phytonutrient called carotenoids than those without the disease.

The carotenoids, which are found in large amounts in most leafy greens, are like bodyguards against cancer-causing agents, explains Frederick Khachik, Ph.D., research chemist at the Food Composition Laboratory at the U.S. Department of Agriculture in Beltsville, Maryland. Scientists believe that certain cancers are brought on by the constant onslaught of free radicals, the renegade molecules that attack our bodies' healthy cells. Carotenoids counteract free radicals by acting as antioxidants, meaning that they step between the free radicals and our bodies' cells, neutralizing them before they can do damage.

While all leafy greens are rich in carotenoids, the granddaddy is spinach, with a half-cup providing 1 milligram of beta-carotene.

Saving Eyes

Carrots must be good for your eyes, the old joke has it, since you never see a rabbit wearing glasses. According to research, it's probably not only carrots that are good for the eyes but also all the leafy greens that Peter and his cottontailed friends munch.

In one study, scientists from the Massachusetts Eye and Ear Infirmary in Boston compared the diets of more than 350 people with advanced age-related macular degeneration—the leading cause of irreversible vision loss among older adults—with the diets of more than 500 people without the disease. They found that people who ate the most leafy green vegetables—particularly, spinach and collard greens—were 43 percent less likely to get macular degeneration than those who ate them less frequently.

Experts believe that carotenoids protect the eyes in much the same way as they work against cancer: by acting as antioxidants and neutralizing tissue-damaging free radicals before they harm the body—in this case, the macular region of the eye.

Mineral Imports

In some parts of the world, like rural China, where vegetarianism is a way of life, people meet their daily calcium needs not by drinking milk but by eating greens. In fact, 1 cup of turnip or dandelion greens can deliver about 172 milligrams of calcium, 17 percent of the DV. That's more than you'd get from a half-cup of fat-free milk.

The only problem with getting calcium from leafy green vegetables is that some of them contain high amounts of oxalates—compounds that block calcium absorption, says Dr. Liebman. "Spinach, Swiss chard, collards, and beet greens

NATURALFACT

Don't depend on the iceberg lettuce that is featured at many salad bars for much nutrition help. Romaine lettuce has twice as much calcium and iron and eight times as much vitamin A and vitamin C as iceberg lettuce.

have the most oxalates, so don't consider these a source of calcium," he says. "The others are fine. Research has shown that the calcium in kale is particularly well-absorbed."

Iron is another mineral found in many greens, especially spinach and Swiss chard. A half-cup of boiled spinach has 3 milligrams of iron, 20 percent of the Recommended Dietary Allowance (RDA) for women and 30 percent of the RDA for men. Swiss chard provides 2 milligrams, which is 13 percent of the RDA for women and 30 percent of the RDA for men.

Leafy greens also contain ample amounts of vitamin C, which help the body absorb the iron. The green giants of vitamin C are chicory (a half-cup serving has 22 milligrams, 37 percent of the DV) and beet and mustard greens, both of which provide almost 18 milligrams, 30 percent of the DV. In addition, beet greens and spinach are rich sources of riboflavin, a B vitamin that is essential for tissue growth and repair as well as helping your body convert other nutrients into usable forms. A half-cup of cooked spinach or beet greens provides 0.2 milligram of riboflavin, 12 percent of the DV.

Sesame Spinach

Give the heave-ho to canned spinach and try this fresh low-sodium side dish instead.

1 tsp canola oil
1 small onion, chopped

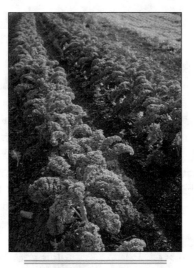

> ## "These are the most nutrient-dense foods that we have available."
>
> —Michael Liebman, Ph.D., professor of human nutrition at the University of Wyoming in Laramie.

1½ pounds spinach, stems removed
¼ cup reduced-fat chicken broth
1 tsp sesame seeds, toasted

In a 4-quart pot over medium-high heat, warm the oil. Add the onion and sauté for 3 to 4 minutes, or until tender. Stir in the spinach and broth and bring to a boil. Reduce the heat, cover, and cook for 2 to 3 minutes, or until the spinach is tender. Sprinkle with the sesame seeds before serving.

Makes 4 servings

Per serving: 62 calories, 6 g protein, 9 g carbohydrates, 2 g fat, 0.5 g saturated fat, 0 mg cholesterol, 5 g dietary fiber, 164 mg sodium

Shrimp and Spinach Toss

Here's a sophisticated combination of flavors that's as tasty as it is healthy.

1 medium onion, thinly sliced
3 garlic cloves, minced
1 Tbsp olive oil
6 cups coarsely chopped spinach
½ cup fat-free chicken broth
¾ pound medium shrimp, peeled and deveined, with tails left on
1 cup sliced roasted red peppers
½ tsp freshly ground black pepper
6 ounces spaghetti

In a pot, toss the onion and garlic with the oil. Cover and cook, stirring, over medium heat for 10 minutes, or until the onion is tender.

Add the spinach and broth. Bring to a boil. Cook, tossing often, for 1 to 2 minutes, or until the spinach is tender. Add the shrimp, roasted peppers, and black pepper. Cook, tossing often, for 3 to 4 minutes, or until the shrimp are opaque and cooked through.

Meanwhile, cook the spaghetti according to package directions. Toss the shrimp mixture with the spaghetti and serve.

Makes 4 servings

Per serving: 328 calories, 26 g protein, 42 g carbohydrates, 6 g fat, 1 g saturated fat, 131 mg cholesterol, 4 g dietary fiber, 389 mg sodium

Southern-Style Kale

Two kinds of ground pepper give this zesty dish a pleasant bite. If you prefer less nip, use half the amount of black pepper and eliminate the red pepper.

    1   pound kale, stems removed
    2   cups reduced-fat chicken broth
    1   small onion, chopped
    1   carrot, chopped
    2   garlic cloves, minced
    2   tsp snipped fresh oregano or ½ tsp dried
    1   tsp canola oil
    ½   tsp black pepper
    ⅛   tsp ground red pepper
    2   potatoes, peeled and quartered

Tear the kale into bite-size pieces. In a large pot or Dutch oven, combine the kale, broth, onion, carrot, garlic, oregano, oil, black pepper, and red pepper. Bring the mixture to a boil over high heat, stirring occasionally.

Add the potatoes. Reduce the heat to

Roll Away the Stone

Popeye probably never had kidney stones because if he had, he wouldn't have kept downing all those cans of spinach.

Spinach, along with Swiss chard and beet greens, contains high amounts of oxalates, acids that the body cannot process and that are passed through the urine. For people who are sensitive to ox-alates, eating too many of these greens can cause painful kidney stones to form. So if you're prone to stones, says Michael Liebman, Ph.D., professor of human nutri-tion at the University of Wyoming in Laramie, forget the chard, spinach, and beet greens. In-stead, choose among other leafy greens, such as dandelion greens, mustard greens, turnip, greens and chicory greens.

medium. Cover and cook, stirring occasion-ally, for 30 minutes, or until the vegetables are tender.

Makes 4 servings

Per serving: 153 calories, 7 g protein, 30 g carbohydrates, 2.5 g fat, 0.5 g saturated fat, 0 mg cholesterol, 6 g dietary fiber, 296 mg sodium

Variation: Substitute olive oil for the canola. Replace the ground red pepper with hot-pepper sauce.

NATURAL HEALING IN THE FUTURE

Heart Disease, Aisle Five

Clare M. Hasler, Ph.D., is the executive director of the Functional Foods for Health Program at the University of Illinois, the nation's first and only program devoted to the study of how foods fight disease. She is a member of the American Nutraceutical Association, the American Institute of Nutritional Sciences,

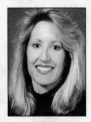

the American Association for Cancer Research, and the Society of Toxicology. There is probably no researcher more qualified to address the future of food than Dr. Hasler.

Q: What have been key significant developments in food research in the past decade?

A: The first thing I'd mention is the huge shift away from thinking that the role of nutrition is to remedy diet deficiencies. Now, when we think about nutrition, we think in terms of how it can bring about optimal health.

For example, we don't just take vitamin C to prevent scurvy, which occurs when you suffer from a chronic deficiency of vitamin C. Today, we take C to cover that deficiency "base," sure, but also to decrease our incidence of colds and to protect us against cataracts in old age. We've gone from thinking about deficiencies to thinking about preventing chronic diseases.

The second trend I see is a move toward more research on nonnutritive substances in foods. By nutrients I mean protein, carbohy-

drates, fat, vitamins, minerals, and water—these keep you alive. Whereas nonnutritive substances—and I'm talking about phytonutrients such as lutein and lycopene, herbs, and many other substances—are not necessary for life. However, they may be necessary for a *healthy* life. A cancer-free life, for example. A lot more research has been focusing on these nonnutritive substances in the past 5 to 10 years. And I see this as a good thing. It parallels the shift in the medical and health-care fields from treatment to prevention.

Q: What products might consumers expect to see on the grocery shelves in the new millennium?

A: Since people are living longer, the average age of our population is increasing. This means that more research money will be aimed at problems that afflict older Americans—heart disease, cancer, osteoporosis, and several others. I believe the day is coming soon when grocery stores will be organized by special needs. You'll be able to walk into a store and go to a kiosk where you key in data on yourself. From this you will get a risk profile. Based on your risk, you will be sent to, for example, aisle B for cardiovascular disease. And aisle B will be stocked with foods that protect against heart disease.

Q: It makes so much sense, it's surprising it hasn't happened already.

A: Not yet, but it will. I'm sure of it. The baby boomers will see to that.

Herbs are usually safer than prescription drugs, with no side effects. They also help us reconnect with nature.

Part Five

Modern
Herbal
Cures

For centuries, the healing powers of herbs have been mainstays of personal health. Now you can put that ancient wisdom to work in your home.

Chapter 11

Herbal Remedies That Work

Here is your easy guide to curing common health problems, naturally

Most of us learned as school children that Christopher Columbus was looking for "spices" when he stumbled on the big chunk of land that would come to be called America. But think about that for a second: Would Columbus and his rivals really have spent years of their lives risking death in the briny deep for something that made their food taste a little tangier?

Probably not. They might, however, have gone to all that trouble if they were also looking for herbs. Healing herbs, to be exact. Which is precisely what they were looking for, in addition to the spices.

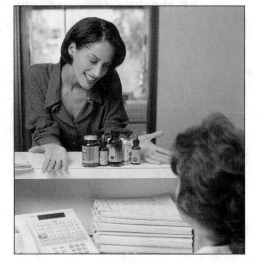

Today, we don't have to cross oceans to get herbal remedies. Even the rarest herbs are available through the mail or at the local health food store. But availability isn't enough.

Herbal Wisdom Preserved

Knowing how to use herbs is as important as being able to get our hands on them readily.

Herbalism is an ancient art, for a long time forgotten by all but a select few.

Now you can share the herbalist's wisdom. We've asked dozens of the most qualified herbalists and alternative medicine experts to

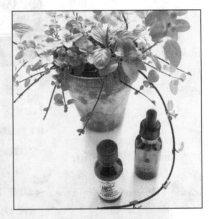

Be Herb Smart

Although herbs are generally far safer than prescription drugs, they are medicine and should be used accordingly.

Check with your doctor before taking herbs in place of your prescription medications, especially those for chronic conditions such as diabetes or high blood pressure. Also, get your physician's stamp of approval before you add herbs to your medications in the hope of achieving better results. If you're taking a digitalis-type medication for your heart condition, for example, you could develop serious problems by adding hawthorn.

Herbs rarely cause side effects. But if you suddenly develop skin rashes, headaches, diarrhea, or nausea lasting longer than 2 days, your body might be telling you that it doesn't want these substances. Work with a health practitioner qualified in the use of herbal remedies to determine if these symptoms mean that you need to reduce the amount of herb, change the specific formula, or switch to a different formula altogether.

Two special cautions:

• Stop using herbs as soon as you know you are pregnant.

• Practice extra caution when using essential oils—extracts distilled from the roots, resins, bark, wood, fruit, leaves, and flowers of plants. Potent and complex, essential oils should never be swallowed because ingesting even a few drops can be toxic. They are best used in diluted form, either externally as massage oils or inhaled. With the exception of lavender, essential oils applied full-strength to the skin can cause burning and irritation.

share with us their top healing secrets for dozens of the most common health problems. Their answers follow. The remedies they recommend are readily available at health food stores, from mail-order catalogs, and in some cases, even at your local supermarket or drugstore. They were selected because they are easy to use or simple to make. More important, when used properly, they're safe and usually side-effect free. (For more detailed safety precautions, see "Be Herb Smart" on page 103. For safety recommendations on the use of specific herbs, oils, and tinctures, see the chart on page 223.)

Let the healing begin.

‖ Allergies

In essence, allergies are overreactions. Your immune system identifies everyday substances like dust mites, pet dander, and mold spores as dangerous invaders. It then goes into overdrive trying to fight the invasion, which is why you end up with all those familiar symptoms, from sniffles and skin inflammation to indigestion and headaches.

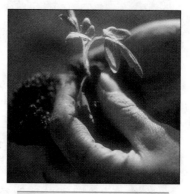

"I think that people have an inherent trust in nature. Even people who are just coming to herbs, who may be a little nervous about taking something that doesn't come from a pharmacy, want to trust that inborn sense that nature is the right place to start the healing process."

—Cascade Anderson Geller, herbal educator and practitioner in Portland, Oregon

Standard over-the-counter decongestants and antihistamines are effective remedies, but they also have side effects: drowsiness, insomnia, even raised blood pressure in some people. Herbalists have other ideas.

Eyebright. If allergies leave you with weepy, watery eyes, turn to eyebright. Herbalists say that this herb naturally tones and strengthens the ocular membranes behind the eyes and can stop eye watering. Drink 1 to 4 milligrams of eyebright as a tincture three times a day, as needed.

Ginkgo. Used by some natural healers specifically for allergies, ginkgo contains compounds called ginkgolides that may counter spasms of the bronchial muscles when your immune system is exposed to an allergen like pollen or animal dander. As a result, you can breathe comfortably instead of wheezing. Take 20 to 30 drops of gingko tincture up to four times a day. You can dilute the dose in water, juice, or herbal tea.

Garlic. Garlic contains high concentrations of the compound quercetin, noted for reducing the severity of inflammatory reactions. If you have allergies, add generous amounts of garlic to your meals.

‖ Arthritis

More than a hundred forms of arthritis exist. Degenerative joint disease (osteoarthritis) is commonly called the wear-and-tear arthritis because it occurs when the cartilage within the joints breaks down. The cause of rheumatoid arthritis, another common form, is unknown, but experts speculate that it may occur when the immune system attacks normal joint tissues.

Mainstream doctors tend to treat arthritis with drugs like steroids, nonsteroidal anti-inflammatory drugs, and sometimes surgery, but herbal medicine has some wonderful alternative answers.

White willow bark. White willow was the original source of aspirin, but it's not as irritating to the stomach, and a cup of white willow bark tea can do wonders to relieve the inflammation in a sore joint. To make the tea, steep 1 teaspoon of white willow bark in a cup of boiling water, covered, for 15 minutes. Strain out the bark and drink a cup three times a day.

NATURALFACT

Thirty to forty percent of all prescription medicines are derived from plants or were developed from clues about the way plant substances affect the human body.

Burdock and dandelion. Herbalists believe that if you stimulate liver function and improve the flow of bile, it helps improve arthritis. Dandelion and burdock will do just that. To make an arthritis-soothing tea, boil 1 teaspoon each of dried dandelion root and dried burdock root in 3 cups of water for 5 minutes, then sip it throughout the day. Drink it daily until you notice some improvement. Be prepared, though—the tea tastes bitter. You can add a little honey to make it more palatable.

Agrimony. Agrimony is known as a traditional medicine for what people used to call rheumatism. It's a great herb for reducing pain and inflammation. Herbal textbooks recommend taking 1 to 3 drops of tincture one to three times a day as needed for pain.

‖ Asthma

Classic triggers of asthma attacks include exposure to air pollutants, pet dander, pollen, or mold. A

Get a Leg Up

If you have knee or hip arthritis aches, ask your doctor to check the length of both your legs. Nearly 20 percent of people with hip arthritis have a 2 centimeter (about ¾ inch) or greater discrepancy in leg lengths, according to a report at the University of North Carolina School of Medicine in Chapel Hill. Unequal leg lengths can easily be remedied with shoe lifts.

bad cold, exercise, stress, crying, anger, hormone fluctuations during menstruation or pregnancy, and even hearty laughter can also set them off.

No matter the cause, what happens inside your lungs during an asthma attack is the same: The tubes that allow oxygen to pass into your lungs tighten and swell. At the same time, these passages produce mucus, which further clogs airways. Breathing becomes difficult, and you may wheeze, cough, or feel tightness in your chest.

Asthma should never be ignored. It's important to see your doctor for a treatment plan. She's likely to prescribe drugs that

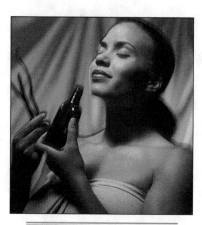

> **"The heaving of my lungs provokes me to ridiculous smiling."**
>
> —William Shakespeare

will quickly relax constricted breathing passages and reduce inflammation. You should never stop taking your asthma medication without your doctor's approval, and always check with your doctor before you take herbs along with any prescription medication. That said, you can reduce your dependence on these medications and breathe easier with the following herbal treatments.

Licorice. Licorice contains a variety of compounds that can lessen the severity of asthma attacks.

To make a cough-soothing licorice tea, simmer a heaping tablespoon of licorice root,

Lavender Essential Oil

Our bodies need to perspire, but sweat can contribute to nasty things like body odor and athlete's foot. Here's how to make an herbal powder that can help both conditions. It contains tea tree oil and powdered ginger, both of which have antiseptic and antifungal action. (If you're making a body powder, you may prefer to use lavender essential oil in place of the tea tree oil; it has a little less antiseptic power, but more fragrance.)

In a large jar, combine ½ cup powdered arrowroot, ½ cup cosmetic clay, and 2 tablespoons powdered ginger. Cover, then shake to mix. Add 20 drops of tea tree oil (or lavender essential oil) and shake again. (You may want to sift the powder through a fine mesh strainer to break up any drops of oil.) Store in a covered, dark glass jar.

Apply as needed to feet or body. Stored in a cool, dry place, the powder will keep indefinitely.

sliced or powdered, in boiling water for 10 minutes. Strain and drink hot daily. To save time, make 3 cups at once and reheat later in the microwave. Or, take 1 table-spoon of licorice tincture daily.

Caution: Licorice is not rec-ommended for long-term use, es-pecially for people with high blood pressure, as it has been known to raise blood pressure when used for long periods.

Ginkgo. Ginkgo interferes with a protein in the blood re-sponsible for causing spasms in bronchial tubes. For best results, take 60 to 240 milligrams of standardized gingko extract a day. If you exceed that amount, you risk diarrhea, irritability, and restlessness.

Evening primrose. Evening primrose oil may reduce the airway inflammation associ-ated with asthma. Experts recommend two 500-milligram capsules of evening primrose oil three times a day.

Athlete's Foot

Athlete's foot is a fungus, and like most fungal critters, it feels at home in moist, damp condi-tions—inside shoes and socks, for example, espe-cially when they don't get washed. To avoid developing athlete's foot in the first place, you need to wash your socks regularly and rotate the shoes you wear (athletic and otherwise) so that each pair has a chance to dry and air out. If you already have athlete's foot, however, there are

NATURALFACT

Ten percent of U.S. adults currently have back pain. Back pain is the number two reason (after fatigue) why people visit a medical clinic.

some herbal remedies that can help you commit fungicide.

Tea tree oil. Tea tree oil is so effective a fungus fighter that it has helped overcome cases of athlete's foot that resisted conven-tional medicines for years. Mix an antifungal soak by diluting 5 to 7 drops of tea tree essential oil in 4 ounces of warm water in a tub large enough to accommodate your feet. Double the recipe if you need more water to cover the affected area. Soak once a day for 20 minutes. Within 5 days, you should see a dramatic improvement. If not, it's fine to increase the soaks up to three times a day. Dry off with a clean towel after each soaking.

Calendula. Research suggests that calen-dula helps promote the growth of new skin cells. So, after you've used an antifungal foot bath for 3 days, begin applying a light calendula cream or salve after each soak.

Lavender. A good way to keep fungus from coming back, or to prevent it growing in the first place, is to make some homemade lavender foot powder. Grind ¼ cup of lavender flowers in a coffee mill or food processor, then mix with ½ cup powdered bentonite clay. Sprinkle it onto your clean, dry feet or right into your clean cotton socks.

Back Pain

Your back is a large expanse of muscles, nerves, tendons, and numerous other elements, all supported on an array of intricately sculpted bones called the vertebrae. Given the complexity of this setup, it is no wonder that most of us will experience a bout of back pain at least once in a lifetime, if not more often. See your doctor if your back pain persists for longer than a week. In the meantime, here are some herbal remedies that may help ease the ache.

Valerian. Although it's best known as a mild sedative to treat insomnia, the soothing qualities of valerian can provide pain relief for a backache triggered by overworked, spastic muscles. That's because muscles in pain tend to tense up. Relaxed muscles, on the other hand, tend to heal faster. Valerian can help your muscles relax. Take two 250-milligram capsules four times a day or 20 drops of tincture every 2 hours.

Other herbs that can help promote muscle relaxation are passionflower, hops, and skullcap. Drink any of them as teas or use as tinctures, putting 30 to 45 drops in 1 cup of water.

Bromelain. Bromelain, an enzyme derived from the stem and leaves of the pineapple

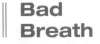

NATURALFACT

Adverse drug reactions are believed to be the 4th to 6th leading cause of death of all Americans.

plant, promotes circulation and helps your body reabsorb all the by-products of inflammation. The result: You heal faster.

Take 500 milligrams three to four times a day an hour after meals. Bromelain strength is standardized in milk-clotting units (mcu) or gelatin-dissolving units (gdu). Look for a product that has a strength between 1,200 and 2,400 mcu or between 720 and 1,440 gdu.

Arnica. Known as the mountain daisy, arnica has pain-relieving, antiseptic, and anti-inflammatory properties. Arnica oil is available at your local health food store, and it can be rubbed on an aching back for soothing relief.

Bad Breath

Everyone's breath needs help now and then. Happily, herbal breath refreshers are plentiful and easy to use. Keep in mind, however, that a persistent odor can signal a more serious

Make It Yourself

Here's an herbal mouthwash recipe from one of America's foremost authorities on folk medicine, John Heinerman, Ph.D., director of the Anthropological Research Center in Salt Lake City.

Combine 10½ tablespoons ground cinnamon per 1¼ cups 100 proof vodka. Put in a bottle and let set for 2 weeks, shaking twice daily (morning and evening). After 2 weeks, strain through cheesecloth or a coffee filter and store in a suitable bottle. Swish and gargle for 1 minute.

Note: Apple cider vinegar may be used as a substitute for the vodka.

A Question of Perception

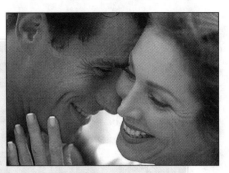

Scientists who study chronic bad breath, known as halitosis, report that people have wildly mistaken ideas about how pleasant or unpleasant their own breath is. One study found that women tend to worry about bad breath when they shouldn't, while men are more likely to think they smell sweet as a rose when they don't.

gum or intestinal problem. If you don't see any improvement within 4 days, or if the odor is really bad, see a dentist or medical doctor.

Cinnamon and clove. These two herbs are potent antiseptics that, when combined in an herbal tea, can wipe out the bacteria that cause bad breath. Just add 4 whole cloves and 2 tablespoons broken-up cinnamon sticks (available in grocery stores) to 1 quart water. Bring to a boil, cover, and simmer for 5 minutes. Set aside and let steep, covered, for 20 minutes. Strain and drink a cup for long-lasting fresh breath.

Parsley. Chlorophyll's powerful germ-fighting forces can tame even the fiercest breath. Simply chew on 10 to 15 parsley sprigs (the ones you find in the grocery store produce section) with all of your teeth, especially the back molars. Grind slowly and methodically for a few minutes, allowing the parsley to mix with saliva until there's nothing left to swallow.

Peppermint tea. The aromatic oil that gives peppermint its distinctive flavor and smell is a potent antiseptic that can kill germs that cause bad breath. Drink a cup of peppermint tea whenever you feel the need.

‖ Bronchitis

When a virus or bacteria makes its way into the lungs, the bronchial tubes respond by swelling and filling with mucus. As the tubes thicken, the tiny airways become even tinier, and soon you have uncontrollable spells of coughing and hacking, your body's way of clearing out the mucus.

Chronic coughs need to be investigated by a doctor, but for coughs that come with a cold, use your standard cold remedies (including plenty of water and plenty of rest) and try these herbal cough suppressors.

Eucalyptus. Buy essential oil of eucalyptus at the health food store and dilute 2 drops of it in 1 ounce of almond oil or castor oil. Rub the resulting mixture liberally on your chest, cover the oiled area with plastic wrap, then a thin towel, and apply a heating pad to help the oil penetrate your tissues.

For a soothing steam inhalation, put a few drops of eucalyptus oil in a pan of water and heat to boiling. Then remove the water from the stove and inhale the steam deeply, being careful not to let the steam burn your face or your nostrils.

Mullein. This is a traditional remedy for respiratory or bronchial coughs. Take a dropperful of mullein tincture in a little warm water every 4 hours while you're ill.

Garlic. Herbal wisdom says that this odoriferous herb contains powerful antibiotic compounds that are actually excreted through the lungs, so they help treat bronchial conditions from the inside out. Try eating a clove of raw garlic during the day or taking an enteric-coated garlic capsule or tablet.

NATURALFACT

If you have a canker sore, avoid acid-forming foods such as citrus, sugar, alcohol, and chewing gum.

‖ Bruises

When you bang your shin, small blood vessels just beneath the surface of the skin break open, releasing blood. The blood seeps out of the injured vessel, making the skin around it black and blue.

In addition to the traditional first-aid remedies—applying an ice pack and keeping the injured limb elevated—here are some herbal remedies that can help move things along.

Witch hazel or oil of lavender. For quick relief, apply either of these immediately to the bruise. Lavender helps lessen the flow of pain impulses, while witch hazel contains natural astringents that help shrink swollen and inflamed tissue.

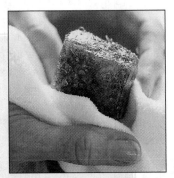

An Icy Treatment

Parsley has a traditional reputation for dispelling black-and-blue marks, and ice can prevent swelling. Combine the two, and you'll have a bruise remedy at the ready in your freezer, says herbalist Sharleen Andrews-Miller, faculty member at the National College of Naturopathic Medicine in Portland, Oregon, and associate medicinary director at the college's public clinic.

"Just whirl a handful of parsley and about a quarter-cup of water in a blender or food processor until it looks like slush. Then fill ice-cube trays half-full," she suggests. "Wrap frozen cubes in gauze or thin cloth and apply to bruised spots as needed. Parsley ice cubes also work well for cooling minor burns."

Arnica. Known as mountain daisy, arnica is a big ally to bruised skin because of its pain-fighting, antiseptic, and anti-inflammatory qualities. Use arnica in a cream or oil form applied directly on the bruised area at least once a day until discoloration disappears. If using a cream, select one that contains up to 15 percent arnica oil for best results.

Bromelain. This pineapple extract contains a protein-digesting enzyme that works to decrease inflammation in bruises. Take 500 milligrams of bromelain three times a day between meals. Look for capsules with a potency of 2,400 mcu.

‖ Burns

One and a half million of us are burned each year, most frequently in accidents at home. Fortunately, most burns and scalds are minor and can be treated safely without a trip to the emergency room. If your burn is so severe that the skin is grayish and numb, you should get to a doctor or an emergency room right away. Also see a doctor if you have blistery burns over a skin area wider than your fist, or if these burns are on your face, hands, feet, groin area, or buttocks. Otherwise, by stocking a few herbal remedies, you can turn your kitchen into a treatment center for minor burns.

For minor burns or scalds, first, cool the spot by running cold water over it for as long as it takes to ease the pain—at least 5 minutes. Then, gently pat the burn dry and proceed with these herbal burn and scald soothers:

Aloe. Aloe gel is herbalists' top recommendation for burn relief because it helps keep burned tissues moist, which is key for healing.

Butter Not

People have long put butter on minor burns to keep them moist, but it's safer to use other salves, says David Seligman, M.D., a pediatrician in Holyoke, Massachusetts. "Butter is a good medium for bacteria to grow in," he says. "Put butter on a burn, and you're asking for an infection."

If you have an aloe plant, cut off an outer leaf, then slit it open lengthwise. Squeeze or scrape out the gel and smear it on the burn. Apply several times a day until the burn heals. If you don't have a plant, or if you have a small one and need more gel than it can provide, you can purchase aloe vera gel at health food stores.

Calendula and comfrey. Once a minor burn has started healing, a calendula-and-comfrey salve will help the skin heal with less scarring. Both herbs have traditional reputations as skin menders.

Again, this is a remedy for minor burns and scalds, *not* for any burn that shows signs of infection, such as redness, puffiness, or oozing. Comfrey promotes such quick cell regeneration that the surface of the burn could heal, leaving damaged skin underneath.

‖ Canker Sores

Stress, hormonal fluctuations, and lowered immunity have often been blamed for causing canker sores, but no one is really sure what makes them sprout. (Don't confuse canker sores with cold sores. The latter are an unwelcome gift of the herpes simplex type 1 virus.) While canker sores usually go away in their own time, they can be acutely painful. Here are some ways to hurry their departure.

Tea tree oil. This is an antiseptic oil, derived from the Australian tea tree, which is available in health food stores. Be careful; it's strong stuff. Apply 1 drop and 1 drop only directly to the sore to help guard against further infection. Let it sit on the sore and dissipate in your mouth, as opposed to quickly swallowing.

Echinacea. Canker sores can crop up when your immunity drops down. Echinacea will help boost your immune system back into fighting shape. Take 200 milligrams three times a day.

Another option is to add a dropperful or two of echinacea tincture to a glass of water and rinse your mouth two or three times a day.

Grapefruit. Eating fresh grapefruit might be torture if you have a canker sore. Grapefruit extract, on the other hand, can work wonders. Buy some at a health food store and dab a drop right on the sore a few times a day. Or, add 5 drops to a glass of water and swish the

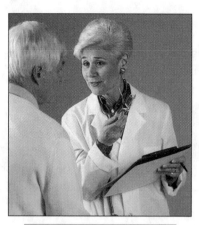

"You should see a doctor if any of your symptoms last more than 5 days. Other than that, there's really nothing a doctor can do, because colds and the flu cannot be helped by antibiotics."

—David Rooney, M.D., a family physician with Southern Chester County Family Practice Associates in Oxford, Pennsylvania

solution around in your mouth three times a day.

‖ Cavities

How can you maintain a healthy, attractive smile? No news here. Brush and floss daily, don't overindulge in sweets, and report faithfully for dental checkups twice a year. Beyond these basic strategies, however, herbalists have plenty of botanical remedies to help cope with common dental concerns.

Bloodroot. To keep sticky dental plaque from adhering to your teeth, look for toothpastes and mouthwashes that contain bloodroot. Studies have shown that dental-care products containing this herb can reduce plaque buildup on teeth within as little as 8 days. Bloodroot contains an alkaloid that chemically binds to dental plaque and keeps it from sticking to your teeth.

Green tea. To prevent cavities, switch your drink of choice from diet soda to herbal tea. Sodas eat away at your tooth enamel. Green and black teas, by contrast, contain a generous amount of tooth-preserving fluoride. Four cups of tea per day—hot or cold—will give you all the fluoride you need.

Clove oil. Once you have a toothache, you need to see a dentist. But to minimize discomfort in the meantime, rub a drop of essential oil of clove directly on your aching tooth.

‖ Colds

If you wonder why you get so many colds, consider the fact that there are roughly 200 known cold viruses, each with a slightly different effect on your body. Your body's response doesn't vary much between each virus, though, which is why they are all lumped together under one name: the common cold.

Cold viruses enter your body via the air (someone has coughed or sneezed nearby) or your fingers (you touched a surface where a cold virus was sitting, and then touched your eyes, nose, or mouth). Once in your body, the virus latches on to mucous membranes that line your nose and throat and quickly multiply.

In addition to the usual cold prescriptions—rest, drink fluids, and take vitamin C—

NATURALFACT

People are most infectious during the first 3 days that they have a cold.

herbs can help catch and kill a cold virus before you can say "Gesundheit."

Echinacea. Studies have shown that this centuries-old remedy is a powerhouse when it comes to bolstering immunity. That's because it stimulates the production of white blood cells, which in turn kill viruses. The moment you feel sneezy and stuffy, take two 200-milligram capsules of echinacea every 2 hours for the first 24 hours. On the second day, take the same dosage every 4 hours, and then every 6 hours after that while cold symptoms last.

You can also use echinacea in tincture form. Place 40 drops in a 6- to 8-ounce glass of water or juice. Repeat the dose every 2 hours. On the second day, drink the mixture every 4 hours, and every 6 hours thereafter.

Eucalyptus. Inhaling the steam from eucalyptus essential oil and water can unstuff a nose naturally and pleasantly. Put 10 to 15 drops of eucalyptus oil in a pan of water, heat to boiling, and remove the pan from the stove.

Shake a Stuffy Nose

A great remedy for a stuffy nose is as near as your kitchen spice rack. "Both red and black pepper dilate blood vessels in the nose and stimulate secretions, which help drain sinuses," says Mark Stengler, N.D., a naturopathic doctor and author of *The Natural Physician.*

To clear up your stuffy nose, simply spice up your food by sprinkling red (sometimes called cayenne) or black pepper (ground or flaked), to taste, on meals. These spices blend especially well with salads, soups, chicken, and pasta.

Covering your head with a towel and leaning over the pan, close enough to feel the steam (about 12 inches away), but not so close that it burns, inhale the steam through your nostrils and blow your nose frequently. Repeat the steam inhalation three or four times daily. Be careful not to let the steam burn your face or sinuses while taking this steam bath.

Astragalus root. This herb has been used for thousands of years in China to enhance immunity, and modern science has affirmed that it enhances several of the body's key disease-fighting functions. To stamp out a cold or flu in its earliest stages, take one 500-milligram capsule of astragalus four times a day until symptoms disappear. Then take one 500-milligram capsule twice a day for 7 days to prevent a relapse.

‖ Constipation

When our digestive machinery is working smoothly, elimination is something we don't need to think about. When it's not working smoothly, it's something we think about a lot. How to get things moving again? The following herbal remedies can help.

Garlic. Sometimes certain strains of bacteria in the colon can cause changes in stool consistency. Garlic is a bacteria-killer, and it can help soften stools by increasing bile flow to the intestines. Take two capsules of garlic (300 to 400 milligrams per capsule) twice a day with your largest meals.

Cascara sagrada. This is a popular, time-tested laxative herb used in dozens of over-the-counter constipation remedies. Take ½ teaspoon at bedtime. But don't use it regularly; your colon may become dependent on it.

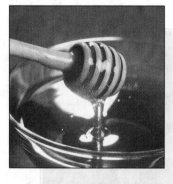

Sweet Treatment

Experts believe that honey may accelerate healing in cuts and scrapes that aren't infected. The sticky stuff covers the wound and starves any bacteria so they stop growing, says Manfred Kroger, Ph.D., professor of food science at Pennsylvania State University in State College. This serves as a protective barrier against new bacteria. Enzymes in honey may also promote skin growth.

To apply, wash the wound thoroughly with soap and water. Smooth a dab of pasteurized honey—the kind from the grocery store—over the wound and cover with a bandage. Repeat three times a day. Watch for signs of infection and do not use honey on cuts that require a doctor's attention.

Dandelion root, gentian root, and gingerroot. These three herbs, taken together or separately, motivate the stomach to produce acid, the pancreas to produce enzymes, and the liver to produce bile—all key digestive steps. For best results for chronic constipation, take one 250-milligram capsule each of dandelion root, gentian root, and gingerroot with meals until the problem is corrected. If you prefer taking them in tincture form, try 30 drops of each.

Cuts and Scrapes

As protective as your skin is, it is no match for a slip of a kitchen carving knife, the scratch of a cat, or a tumble on a gravel driveway. If the bleeding is hard to control or if you have a cut that is long, wide, and nasty-looking, maintain pressure on the wound and get to an emergency room. Highly contaminated wounds (like those from fishhooks or those with ground-in dirt or manure) may not bleed but are potentially dangerous as well. Don't wait a day "to see what happens." But for minor run-of-the-mill cuts, scrapes, and scratches, open the herbal first-aid kit.

Calendula. Also known as pot marigold, this lovely yellow and orange flowered plant is a natural antiseptic, and it promotes healing. After cleaning the wound with soap and water, put several drops of a non-alcohol-based calendula tincture on the wound two or three times a day.

NATURALFACT

Normally, it takes about 28 days for people to shed old cells from their scalps as new ones push their way to the surface. People who have dandruff shed the cells on their scalps twice as fast as people who don't.

Witch hazel. Witch hazel was long a popular healing herb among native American tribes, and for good reason: Its bark, leaves, and twigs are rich in tannins, making it an excellent astringent that can soothe and protect inflamed, red, itching skin. Use it to cleanse and help mend ragged cuts and scrapes. Avoid using distilled witch hazel water from the drugstore, however; instead, use witch hazel tincture diluted with water to promote more effective healing. Apply to the wound with cotton swabs or a clean cloth.

Myrrh. You know myrrh as one of the gifts that the wise men offered the baby Jesus, but it's also known for its antiseptic powers. Dissolve a teaspoon of myrrh powder (available in health food stores) in a cup of warm water and use that liquid to wash out the cut as promptly as possible.

Dandruff

Skin cells grow, multiply, and die off on your scalp each day. The dead cells flake away invisibly as living cells emerge to the skin's surface, only to repeat the process. When these cells grow and die off too rapidly, however, a flurry of visible dandruff appears.

Despite the embarrassment, dandruff is harmless. Stress, food allergies, yeast infections, and heredity are some of the most common triggers. See your doctor if your flakes are itchy, thick, greasy, and yellow, or if you have dry, thick lesions on your scalp that leave it red and inflamed. Those are signs of more serious skin conditions (dermatitis and psoriasis, respectively).

For run-of-the-mill dandruff, these herbal remedies should end the snowfall:

Rosemary. Make a strong rosemary tea using at least 2 tablespoons of the dried leaf in a cup of boiling water. Steep for at least 20 minutes, then strain and cool. You can also add a few drops of rosemary essential oil to the tea. Use as a hair rinse after shampooing. This rinse will not leave a film on your hair. If you choose to, you can rinse it out after a few minutes, but it is not necessary.

Thyme. You can brew a similar herbal hair tonic using thyme. Boil 4 heaping tablespoons of the dried herb in 2 cups of water in a nonaluminum pot for 10 minutes. Strain it and allow the tea to cool. Pour the brew over damp, freshly shampooed hair and gently massage it into your scalp. Again, there's no need to rinse.

Flaxseed or evening primrose oil. These oils, called essential fatty acids, can prevent the rapid shedding of dead skin cells by promoting the growth of healthier skin tissues from the outset. Take 1 tablespoon daily of the oil or nine 1,000-milligram capsules per day. This isn't a short-term solution: You may need to take these for up to 3 months to see a difference. If there is little or no change after 3 months, switch to a different oil.

‖ Diarrhea

Since we don't usually discuss our bathroom routines with others, you might be surprised to learn that bowel habits vary quite a bit among adults.

You Make the Call

Herbs can work for you in a lot of different ways. Here are the most common methods for utilizing herbal products.

Capsules. Capsules contain herb material that has been crushed into powder and placed in a capsule. Many capsules contain "standardized extracts," meaning that the manufacturer has processed the contents to ensure that they contain a certain amount of one or more of the herb's major active ingredients. This is done to compensate for the wide variability that occurs in the plant's natural state.

Creams. Herbal creams and ointments are available for external use from health food stores and should be applied according to the label instructions.

Essential oils. These are extremely concentrated oils that have been distilled from the flowers,

Some need to defecate three times a day; others, just a few times a week. Diarrhea is loosely defined (if you'll pardon the expression) as stools that are more fluid or more frequent than what is usual for a person.

Any number of things can cause diarrhea, but intestinal infections, bacteria in food or drink, medications, and food allergies (particularly to dairy products) are among the most common triggers. See a doctor if your symptoms last more than 3 days or include fever over leaves, fruit, bark, resins, or roots of plants. More than 1,000 essential oils exist, ranging from the commonplace (peppermint and cinnamon) to exotics, such as tea tree oil from New Zealand, patchouli from Indonesia, and rosewood from India.

Poultices. A poultice is a wad of chopped, fresh, or dried but remoistened plant material that is applied directly to a wound or infection on the skin and usually held in place by a wet dressing that is covered by a bandage.

Teas. Herbal teas can be made from fresh or dried herbs. The latter are more potent because they contain less water, making the active ingredients more concentrated. Herb teas can be either infusions or decoctions. Infusions are made by pouring hot water over a tea bag or loose herbs and steeping for 5 to 10 minutes. Decoctions are made by simmering the herbs in water for 15 to 30 minutes. Decoctions are best for root or stems,

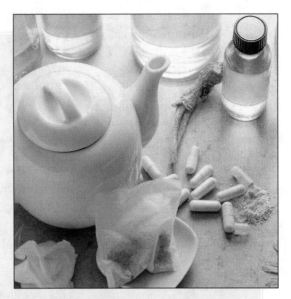

which yield their healing chemicals more reluctantly than do leaves and flowers.

Tinctures. Tinctures, also known as extracts, are made by soaking fresh herbs for days or weeks in alcohol with varying amounts of water. The mixture is then shaken, strained, and bottled for use. Tinctures, which are sold in stores, are usually taken mixed in a little water.

101°F; severe cramps or vomiting; blood, pus, or mucus in your stool. Dehydration (marked by cracked lips or constant, extreme thirst) is also a concern worth checking with your doctor, who can also tell you if any medications you're taking may be the cause of your diarrhea.

Otherwise, add fiber to your diet, stick with the BRAT diet (bananas, rice, applesauce, and toast), and try these herbal remedies.

Goldenseal. This herb contains a chemical called berberine that fights bacteria and

viruses. It also stimulates your immune system. Four times a day, take two 250-milligram capsules of goldenseal or 60 drops of goldenseal tincture in a quarter glass of warm water. If you are sensitive to the alcohol base of the tincture, let the mix sit for 3 minutes, which allows some of the alcohol to evaporate.

Elm and marshmallow. This herbal tandem heals the digestive tract lining. For best results, take two 250-milligram capsules or 60 drops of tincture (in a quarter glass of warm water) of each herb four times a day until the diarrhea subsides.

Cinnamon tea. If your diarrhea is extreme, you may be at risk for dehydration. Cinnamon tea is a natural astringent that can help stop the runs quickly. Mix a tablespoon of dried powdered cinnamon bark into a cup of hot water. Steep for 10 to 15 minutes. Use cinnamon this way only for short periods of time.

NATURALFACT

Among the famous people who have had diabetes: James Cagney, Thomas Edison, Ernest Hemingway, and George Lucas.

cosides. Take 40 milligrams three times a day.

Bay leaf, cinnamon, cloves, and turmeric. Research shows that these spices help the body use insulin more efficiently, and they're easy to use. Simply put a pinch or two each of these herbs into a pot of black tea. Steep for 10 minutes. Pour over a glass of ice and drink.

Ginseng. Taking ginseng may help stabilize type 2 diabetes by helping the body gain greater control of blood sugar levels. Take 200 milligrams in capsule form every day.

Diabetes

If there's one good thing that can be said about type 2 (non-insulin-dependent) diabetes, it's that this disorder usually responds very nicely to diet and lifestyle changes. The nutritional and herbal supplements that are recommended here are no substitute for the fundamental lifestyle changes that can help you control this kind of diabetes. You have to eat right, control your weight, and get regular exercise.

Once those basics have been attended to, however, herbal supplements can complement your efforts. Be sure to talk with your doctor before adding these herbs to your treatment plan and continue monitoring your blood sugar levels carefully. Report any change to your doctor promptly.

Ginkgo. Diabetes can impair circulation, especially in the legs, which is a problem that ginkgo can address. Ginkgo also helps blood circulation to the brain, which requires large amounts of blood sugar. Look for a standardized extract that contains 24 percent ginkgoflavogly-

Earache

There are three primary causes for ear pain: pressure inside the ear, infection, or sudden changes in external air pressure that wrench the eardrum out of position.

Often, nasal congestion is behind those first two causes, while airplanes, elevators, or scuba diving often account for the third. Treatment for an earache depends on the cause. If it's bacterial, a doctor's prescription may be your best choice to kill the infection and reduce pain and inflammation. Also see the doctor if you have truly severe pain, discharge, hearing loss, a fever of 102°F or above, or tenderness when you press the soft areas near your ear, around your jaw, or in the upper neck area. For mild earaches, try these herbal earache erasers.

Garlic and mullein. These herbs are known to be good bacteria fighters, and garlic also helps boost immunity. Place 3 drops of garlic oil and 2 drops of mullein oil directly in the aching ear. Do this three or four times a day until the pain subsides.

Note, however, that you should not put any herbal preparation in your ear if you suspect that your eardrum may have been ruptured.

Echinacea, goldenseal, and garlic. To help fight the germs causing the pain and pressure, give yourself daily doses of these immune-stimulating herbs. Take up to 1,200 milligrams of echinacea in three to six divided doses; 1,800 milligrams of goldenseal in three divided doses, but not for more than a week; and up to 5 milligrams of fresh allicin, the active ingredient in garlic (look for a garlic supplement that says "fresh" on the label).

Another way of boosting your immune system herbally is to make an herbal juice with 30 drops of echinacea and 30 drops of goldenseal tinctures in juice or water.

‖ Eczema

Eczema is an inflammatory skin allergy that can surface on your neck, face, and legs, and within the folds of your elbows, knees, and wrists. Food allergies and stress are among the top contributors to the problem. Laundry detergents, harsh soaps,

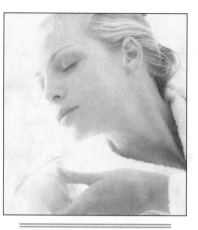

"The goal of good skin care is to maintain the natural barrier your skin provides."

—Mindy Green, professional herbalist

rough and scratchy clothing, dust, pollen, and the dry, cold winter months can also trigger a flare-up.

See your doctor if the eczema is very red, causes severe pain, or drains pus, or if you have a fever—all signs of infection. Since eczema is often spurred by allergies, you may need to take an inventory of your diet and your environment to pinpoint the cause of the reaction. These herbs may also help.

Flaxseed oil or evening primrose oil. These oils, called essential fatty acids, can play a significant role in preventing allergies and inflammation, including skin inflammation. Each day, take 1½ tablespoons of either oil. You can also take 3,000 to 5,000 milligrams of one of these oils in capsule form each day.

Chickweed. This herb is an effective itch soother. Mix 15 drops of chickweed tincture into a 2-inch dollop of moisturizing cream. For best results, rub the cream into the affected area within 3 minutes after you bathe. For longer-term use, blend a tablespoon of the tincture into a cup of moisturizing cream.

Licorice, burdock, and dandelion. A tea made from these three herbs has potent anti-inflammatory and anti-allergenic properties that can help prevent eczema. To make the tea, combine 2 tablespoons each of dried licorice, burdock, and dandelion root in a nonaluminum pot. Pour 3 cups of water into the pot.

Cover it tightly and bring the water to a boil. Let the herbs simmer for 15 to 20 minutes. (If the liquid reduces too much, add enough water so that you end up with three cups of tea.) Strain the tea into a cup and drink.

To get the most benefit, drink a cup of the tea three times a day. If you prefer capsules, take 200 to 500 milligrams of each herb a day.

‖ Fatigue

These days, fatigue is perhaps one of the most common ailments, varying from mild and intermittent to chronic and severe. Sometimes, it's a perfectly healthy response to a demanding day. Other times, an unhealthy diet, lack of exercise, stress, depression, or illness can be the causes.

If you've been so constantly tired for 2 weeks or more that you can't do your normal activities, or if you have muscle aches, nausea, fever, depression, mood swings, or night sweats with your fatigue, see a doctor. But if your fatigue seems to be temporary, here are some herbs that can help you pick up the pace again.

Ginseng. This is the superstar of all energy-boosting herbs. Both Korean ginseng and Siberian ginseng are worth trying. For ginseng tea, place about 1 teaspoon of ginseng in a cup of boiling water. Let it steep for 5 minutes or so, strain, and drink. Stick to one cup a day. If you want to take capsules, follow the specific dosage directions on the product you buy. You may need to take ginseng for a month or more before you see results.

Barley grass or wheat grass. These herbs are full of fatigue-fighting B vitamins and iron. Add them to salads (many organic supermarkets carry these herbs) or buy barley-grass or wheat-grass juice. To fight fatigue, aim to add ½ cup of either grass to your salads each day or drink 8 ounces of juice.

Peppermint. A quick spritz in the face with peppermint water can spring you back to action. Add 15 drops of essential oil of peppermint to an 8-ounce spray bottle of water. Shake well and spray your face and the air around you (with your eyes and mouth closed) whenever you start to drag.

‖ Fever

Fever is your body's way of fighting off infection: it tries to burn out the invaders. You don't want the fever to burn too high, though, or you risk damaging healthy cells. Any fever that's higher

Warming from the Inside

Try this recipe for an herbal tea that will take the chill out of your flu or cold, courtesy of herbalist David Hoffman, of the California Institute of Integral Studies in Santa Rosa.

In a pot or pan, combine 1 ounce (by weight) sliced fresh ginger, 1 broken-up cinnamon stick, 1 teaspoon coriander seeds, 3 cloves, 1 lemon slice, and 1 pint of water. Simmer for 15 minutes and strain. Then drink a hot cupful every 2 hours.

Rub It In

Here's an aromatic rub that can soothe flu symptoms, courtesy of Susanne Wissell, a licensed massage therapist and principal of the Center for Holistic Botanical Studies in Westford, Massachusetts. Pour one ounce of vegetable or almond oil into a small container. Add 11 drops each of eucalyptus and ravensara essential oils, along with 2 drops of cinnamon leaf essential oil. Mix well, then put some drops on your hands and rub the mixture onto your throat and upper chest area. Repeat this treatment throughout the day.

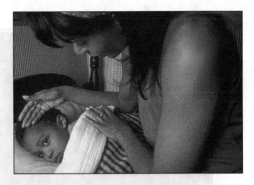

You can also apply this blend all over your body at nighttime. "Put on an old pair of pajamas that you don't mind getting some oil on and get into bed. By the next morning, you should feel fine," says Wissell. Eucalyptus is a natural antiseptic, antibacterial, and antiviral oil; ravensara has abundant antiviral compounds; and cinnamon leaf harbors anti-infection and antiviral properties, she says.

than 103°F or that lasts longer than 48 hours requires prompt medical attention. According to medical experts, though, you do want to let fever run its course so that you can kill the infectious organisms and get well.

While that's happening, apply a cool cloth to your forehead frequently to keep your fever from burning too hot around your head, where it can cause brain damage if unchecked. And take herbs that promote sweating to allow the fever to run its course more quickly and effectively. Be patient when taking them; herbs don't suppress a fever the same way aspirin or other over-the-counter medications do. The goal isn't to cover up the body's natural healing process but to enhance it, which may mean that you'll feel temporarily worse before you feel better.

Here are the herbs that practitioners say best ease you through a bout with fever. As always, check with your health-care practitioner before using herbs as an adjunct to other treatments that he or she may have prescribed.

Elderflower. This herb is good for opening pores and inducing sweat to break a fever. Extract of elderflower also contains compounds that help break up and clear out excess mucus and inflammation that usually accompany fever due to colds and flu.

To make a tea out of dried elderflowers, pour a cup of boiling water over 2 teaspoons of the herb and allow it to steep, covered, for 15 to 20 minutes. Drink it three times a day as needed.

Yarrow. Yarrow contains volatile oils that open your pores and cause profuse sweating to assist in breaking a fever. Make yarrow tea by using 1 tablespoon of the herb per cup of boiling water and steeping it in a covered container for 10 minutes. After drinking a cup or two of this tea, you will start to sweat. Once that happens, you have had enough.

Echinacea. Whenever you have an inflammatory or infectious condition that commonly triggers fever, take echinacea to help boost your immune system. Try taking 30 to 50 drops of liquid echinacea extract in a glass of water, juice, or herbal tea every 2 hours until the fever subsides.

‖ Flu

Like the common cold, influenza viruses are spread by sneezing and coughing. Once these viruses latch on to the mucous membranes in your nose or mouth, a fierce battle ensues. Attempting to rid itself of the virus, your body heats up like a furnace, becomes inflamed in certain places, and produces mucus. As miserable as they are, headache, fatigue, muscle aches, chills, sore throat, dry cough, and congestion all simply reflect that the body is doing its job.

Symptoms should dissipate after 5 to 7 days. If, instead, you are getting weaker, sustaining a temperature above 101°F for more than 48 hours or coughing from more deeply in your chest, see a doctor—pneumonia could be developing. If you have a more run-of-the-mill case, here are some remedies that can help you beat it.

Ginger. Herbal teas are good for a flu-ridden system because warm liquids are soothing, help prevent viruses from reproducing, and even

> **NATURAL**FACT
>
> Did you know that mosquitoes are attracted to foot odor? And to bad breath.

have a mild decongestant effect. Ginger tea in particular is chock-full of antiviral compounds to help fight infection, reduce pain and fever, and suppress coughing. It's also a natural expectorant and a mild sedative that will help you get some rest. To make ginger tea, chop a 1-inch slice of fresh gingerroot into slivers. Place the ginger in a nonaluminum pot. Add 2 cups of water and cover the pot tightly. Simmer for 20 minutes, then strain the tea into a cup. Squeeze in the juice of half a lemon. Add honey to taste.

Elderflower or licorice. These two herbs both have immune-stimulating capabilities. Steeping 2 tablespoons of the dry herb for 10 minutes will bring out all the medicinal qualities of the herbs. Strain before drinking. Sip the tea as needed.

Goldenseal, echinacea, or astragalus. These herbs are powerful allies for your ailing immune system. Take 200 milligrams of any one of these four times a day for 5 to 7 days.

‖ Foot Odor

A pair of feet has approximately 250,000 sweat glands, and they excrete as much as half a pint of moisture each day. Seal all that moisture up inside a pair of shoes and socks, and you have the perfect breeding ground for bacteria and fungi, the sources of foot odor.

The first steps you can take to combat foot odor are to wear clean socks every day and to own more than one pair of shoes so that you can rotate them regularly. While your shoes are airing out, the following herbal remedies may help your feet.

Goldenseal and myrrh. Soaking your feet in a footbath spiced with these herbs will fight both bacteria and fungus. Mix a tablespoon of goldenseal tincture and a tablespoon of myrrh tincture in a half-quart of warm water and soak your feet in it for 5 to 10 minutes once a week. The goldenseal may stain your skin yellow, but it won't hurt you.

Lavender and tea tree. Lavender is among the most skin-friendly of all the healing herbs and thus can help soothe the tissues on your foot that have been irritated by invading bacteria. Meanwhile, the potent antifungal properties of the tea tree oil will send bacteria packing. Try mixing 1 teaspoon of tea tree essential oil with 3 teaspoons of lavender essential oil and rubbing the resulting combination into your feet until it disappears, once in the morning and once at night.

Garlic. Taken internally, garlic can help make your body an inhospitable environment for the types of fungus that create foot odor. Take enough garlic capsules to equal 7,500 micrograms of allicin in three divided doses a day.

‖ Gas

You won't be surprised to hear that flatulence is the result of an overabundance of various forms of gas and bacteria building up in your digestive system. It's quite normal, usually.

If you have sharp pain or tenderness in the

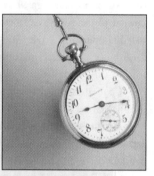

Hypnotherapy

Hypnosis can be just the remedy you need to fend off embarrassing flatulence due to gastrointestinal disorders, says Jack Gerhard, licensed psychologist and hypnosis trainer in Emmaus, Pennsylvania. "I've had patients tell me that because of their gas problem, they can't enjoy life. They get nervous going out to dinner and worry that they won't be near a bathroom at social events," he says. "Hypnosis works with the autonomic nervous system and helps with the digestive process."

Typically, a hypnosis session lasts an hour, with the goal of teaching people self-hypnosis techniques that they can use whenever a need arises. During hypnosis, Gerhard often asks his patients to visualize relaxing images or cool colors. Or, he uses guided imagery to help them confront and then conquer gas-causing foods in their minds. "If you can connect coolness, calmness, and relaxation together, it seems to help take care of stress often associated with gastrointestinal conditions, including gas," he says.

abdomen, see a doctor. This is especially true for "rebound" tenderness, which occurs when you press on your abdomen, release your hand, and have pain after the pressure of your hand is removed. Otherwise, give the following herbal remedies a shot.

Fennel. To ensure that you're free of excess gas, chew ½ teaspoon fennel seeds. Fennel is a carminative, a substance that helps dissipate gas. It also helps correct digestive disturbances by relaxing muscle spasms.

Peppermint. Peppermint, another carminative, soothes digestion and has a reputation for minimizing gas. For best results, pour a cup of just-boiled water over 1 tablespoon of dried peppermint leaves. Steep, covered, for 5 to 10 minutes, then strain and sip. Drink a cup of this tea three or four times daily.

Caution: Avoid drinking this tea if you have esophageal reflux.

Aniseed, basil, and other herbal spices. If you enjoy eating beans or other gas-producing foods, you can tone down the tooting by seasoning your dishes with herbs from the mint and carrot families, herbalists suggest. Keep eating beans, which are an excellent source of high-quality protein, fiber, and other nutrients, but also reach into your spice rack for aniseed, basil, chamomile, cinnamon, garlic, ginger, lemon, onion, oregano, or rosemary—all of which are excellent carminatives.

‖ Headache

Since the causes of headaches vary, so do the cures. Migraines, in particular, are highly indi-

---

NATURALFACT

An estimated 26 million Americans— mostly women— experience migraine headaches.

---

vidualized, so if you experience them, work with your doctor to identify the specific causes and treatment. And see a doctor if your nonmigraine headaches are getting progressively worse in intensity or frequency; if they are accompanied by confusion, memory loss, dizziness, mood swings, double vision, and coordination problems; or if they followed a fall or blow to the head.

Otherwise, here are some natural remedies that may help you cut down your consumption of over-the-counter painkillers.

Feverfew. This herb is so effective at relieving pain caused by inflammation that it was once nicknamed the headache plant. To relieve pain or prevent future headaches, chew two fresh or freeze-dried feverfew leaves. Or, you can make a tea with prepared, dried feverfew using 2 to 3 tablespoons in a cup of hot water. Let the tea steep for at least 10 minutes, then strain it and add sweeteners to suit your taste. For the best effect, have two cups of fresh-brewed tea daily.

Ginkgo. Ginkgo helps increase blood flow to the brain, which may help prevent headaches from starting in the first place. Be patient, however; you may need to take gingko for up to 6 weeks before seeing an effect. Take 40 milligrams of ginkgo three times a day.

Ginger. Ginger tea will help quiet the inflamed blood vessels in your head. It also slows the release of the body's pain-sensitizing chemicals and improves circulation. To make the tea, mix ⅓ teaspoon of powdered ginger or grated fresh ginger in a cup of hot water. Let cool, strain, and drink at the first sign of a headache.

‖ Heartburn

Your esophagus, a long tube that sends food and liquid from the mouth into the stomach, does about the same thing as the drainpipe from your kitchen sink. When all's going well, whatever you eat plunges smoothly toward your stomach. The problem arises—literally—when there is a welling-up from down below, and stomach acid backs up.

See your doctor if your heartburn is severe or prolonged, but easy remedies to calm mild to moderate heartburn are within your reach.

Ginger. Ginger works as an antispasmodic, relaxing the smooth muscle along the walls of the esophagus, which makes it less likely that you'll get a backwash of stomach acid. Be forewarned, however, that some people with sensitive stomachs may find it too spicy. To prevent heartburn, take ginger 20 minutes before a meal, in capsule form or in a cup of ginger tea. Both fresh ginger-root and powdered ginger are available at supermarkets. Another option is ginger tincture: Take between 15 and 60 drops mixed in a little water.

Licorice. Licorice root (sorry, not the stringy candy) prompts the cells that line your

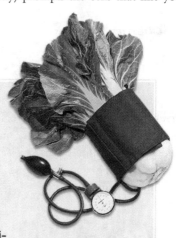

A Heart Warning

Some people think that because some herbal kidney remedies help you excrete water, they're like the diuretics often prescribed for high blood pressure. They're not.

In fact, says top herb expert Varro E. Tyler, Ph.D., Sc.D., distinguished professor emeritus of pharmacognosy and dean emeritus of Purdue University School of Pharmacy and Pharmacal Sciences in West Lafayette, Indiana, they're not diuretics. They're aquaretics, and they don't get at the real cause of high blood pressure. When excessive amounts of electrolytes (especially sodium) are retained in the body, they cause an increase in extracellular fluid and blood (plasma) volume. This places an increased burden on the heart and results in high blood pressure, Dr. Tyler says.

To reduce your blood pressure, you must eliminate both the excess water from the plasma and, even more important, the excess electrolytes. Prescription diuretic drugs are designed to do just that. They act on the kidneys to speed the excretion of both water and electrolytes (aquaretics aid in the excretion of water only), thereby lowering blood pressure. Such drugs are often the first treatment that a physician will prescribe for high blood pressure, according to Dr. Tyler.

stomach to produce mucus, providing a safety coating that protects against your own highly acidic digestive juices. Take two 500-milligram tablets of deglycyrrhizinated licorice root 15 minutes before meals for best results. Make sure that you choose deglycyrrhizinated licorice—it does not contain glycyrrhizin, a substance that can raise blood pressure.

Chamomile. This herb acts as a mild sedative that soothes mucous membranes. To make chamomile tea, add 1 tablespoon of whole dried chamomile flowers to a cup of hot water and steep for 15 minutes. Strain and drink daily. Some herbalists recommend that you keep the teapot and your cup covered so that the vapor can't escape. The volatile oils in the vapor are among chamomile's active ingredients.

High Blood Pressure

If you have high blood pressure, your heart is working harder than it should to pump blood through your system. You may have no idea that this is going on—high blood pressure is a silent destroyer. That's why it's important once you pass your 40th birthday to have your blood pressure checked once a year. Check it in your twenties if there is a family history of heart disease, especially if you don't follow a heart-healthy diet.

Once diagnosed, your doctor can show you plenty of ways to lower blood pressure, including some major lifestyle changes that will probably save your life. As with any form of heart disease,

> **NATURAL**FACT
>
> Studies have shown that people who take garlic can reduce their systolic blood pressure by about 7 percent.

high blood pressure needs professional medical attention. The herbal remedies here should be considered complementary to such treatment and should be checked with your doctor to make sure that the herbs won't interact with any prescription drugs that you might be taking.

Hawthorn. Hawthorn extracts, taken from the berries of the small, thorny English hawthorn tree, contain chemicals called polyphenols that are particularly good for your heart in two ways: First, they dilate blood vessels, particularly coronary arteries, helping reduce blood pressure. Second, they help improve heart function when taken over a long period. Take 250 milligrams of hawthorn in standardized extract form three times a day.

Garlic. This may be the world's most popular medicinal food, for good reason. Among its many health benefits, garlic appears to lower cholesterol in the bloodstream and reduce blood pressure. Eat lots of fresh garlic or take 320 milligrams of garlic extract once or twice a day.

Lemon balm. For high blood pressure triggered by stress, try a daily dose of lemon balm. Take 5 milliliters of lemon balm tincture twice a day for 12 weeks. Then recheck your blood pressure and continue taking as needed. Herbalists say that lemon balm calms as it lifts your spirits, which can translate into lower blood pressure readings.

High Cholesterol

Your heart is an engine, a fist-size machine of chambers and valves that motor your body through its daily activities. In synchronized rhythm, a circuitry of pipes work to deliver the rich fuel of blood throughout your body. But when a fatty substance called cholesterol builds up as plaque along the walls of your arteries, the pipes get clogged. If a blood test reveals that your system is running too rich with cholesterol—specifically, with too much of what is called low-density lipoprotein, or LDL, cholesterol— you run the risk of heart disease.

Heart disease is nothing to fool around with, and a central part of any adult's health regimen is to be tested to make sure your cholesterol level is in line. If it isn't, consult with a doctor, who may recommend a host of remedial actions, from changes in diet and exercise to medications. Herbal remedies can also contribute, but check with your doctor to avoid dangerous drug-herb interactions.

Garlic. Garlic's heart-friendly powers are well-recognized in Europe, where it is an approved remedy for high cholesterol. Cooking garlic destroys much of its healthy properties; aim to eat three raw cloves a day. If you're concerned about the odor, take two odorless garlic supplements three times a day. Look for a brand that says it is standardized to at least 1.3 percent allicin.

> **NATURALFACT**
>
> Ancient Greeks warded off indigestion after a feast by eating ginger wrapped in bread, which is how we got gingerbread.

Flaxseed oil. The oil from these shiny, hard seeds is a rich source of omega-3 fatty acids, a heart-healthy fat that lowers LDL levels and helps prevent blood clots. Take 1½ teaspoons of flaxseed oil every day. One-and-a-half tablespoons of the ground seed is just as omega-rich as the oil, and it also contains fiber. Try adding some to your cereal or yogurt every day.

Guggul. This herb can improve levels of the "good" cholesterol (high-density lipoprotein, or HDL) while simultaneously working to lower levels of LDL cholesterol. Take 500 milligrams in capsule form two or three times a day until your cholesterol normalizes.

‖ Indigestion

We call a lot of things indigestion, but the main cause is what the commercials used to call "excess stomach acid." Probably the best way to combat it, if acid is a problem that you're prone to, is to watch what you eat. Meats, tomato sauce, orange juice, and other acidic

It's Good to Be King

There had to be a reason why all those rich people love caviar. Turns out that the luxury item delivers a burst of omega-3 fats, which are catnip for your heart. Just 1 tablespoon of caviar has 1 gram of hard-to-get omega-3 fats— more than what's in half a can of white tuna. Yet it has only 40 calories and 2.8 grams of total fat. Experts think that omega-3's help your heart muscle beat regularly and thus prevent fatal heart attacks.

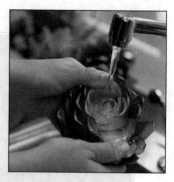

Artichoke for the Stomach

One neglected herbal remedy that may be poised for a takeoff in popularity is a standardized extract of artichoke leaves.

Two placebo-controlled clinical studies have now verified the herb's digestive action, according to one of the world's top herb experts, Varro E. Tyler, Ph.D., Sc.D., distinguished professor emeritus of pharmacognosy and dean emeritus of Purdue University School of Pharmacy and Pharmacal Sciences in West Lafayette, Indiana. Germany's Commission E (that country's equivalent of our FDA and the world's leading authority on herbs) has approved artichoke preparations for the treatment of what are known as dyspeptic complaints, he says. There is also evidence that artichoke has cholesterol-lowering and liver-protecting properties.

foods can be your ticket to stomach trouble. If the problem persists or it's hard to change your diet, herbs can help bring your stomach juices back into balance.

Chamomile. This is one of the most gentle and reliable of the stomach-settling herbs. To make chamomile tea, add 1 full tablespoon of whole dried flowers to 1 cup of hot water and steep for 15 minutes, then strain. If you're prone to indigestion, drink chamomile tea throughout the day to prevent it.

Barberry. The bitter herb barberry can help increase the flow of digestive juices, helping you digest more easily. Try 10 to 20 drops of barberry extract (available at health food stores or by mail order) diluted in about 4 ounces of water 15 to 20 minutes before meals.

Peppermint. This herb calms the nerves in your digestive system. You'll get best results by using fresh or dried leaves to make tea, but store-bought teas can also help. To make the tea, use 1 tablespoon of whole dried leaves (or 2 tablespoons of fresh) or one tea bag per cup of hot water and steep for 10 minutes. Sip slowly. Have a cup in the morning and a cup at night, or more often if you like.

Insect Bites and Stings

Ouch! When mosquitoes bite or bees sting, their attacks can cause redness, itching, swelling, and sometimes, skin infection. Not to mention pain.

If you're stung by a bee, first, safely remove the stinger and sac by scraping them away with your thumbnail or a credit card.

Caution: People allergic to insect venom can develop life-threatening reactions. If you have difficulty breathing or develop hives on your face, arms, legs, or torso, call your local emergency medical number or head to the nearest hospital—pronto. Otherwise, try these simple herbal soothers for fast relief from the pain, itch, swelling, and infection.

Peppermint. For fast relief, rub a tiny droplet of peppermint essential oil into the bull's-eye center of bites and stings. Peppermint essential oil has been used traditionally as an antiseptic and local anesthetic. It cools the area, reducing itching and pain. Thoroughly wash your hands after application so that you won't irritate your eyes.

Calendula. This herb encourages tissue healing and acts as a natural infection-fighting antiseptic. Make a calendula tea using about 1 tablespoon of the dried herb per cup of boiling water. Let it steep for 5 minutes, then strain and let it cool. Dip a cotton ball into the calendula tea and dab it on bites or stings four or five times daily until the skin has healed.

Echinacea. For stubborn bug bites that stay swollen, ease the inflammation with an echinacea poultice. For a small bite, combine 1 teaspoon of echinacea tincture and 1 teaspoon of water with enough bentonite clay to create a thick paste. The clay can be purchased in some

health food stores or herb specialty shops. (You can double this recipe for larger or multiple bites.) Dab the mixture on the bite and cover it with an adhesive strip bandage. Change the dressing twice a day.

‖ Insomnia

Coast to coast, some 20 to 50 million Americans regularly miss out on a good night's rest. Lifestyle adjustments such as avoiding coffee at night and exercising a few times a week can help fight insomnia. So can meditation and progressive relaxation techniques. Natural healers also suggest these good-night herbs for a good night's sleep.

Valerian. This herb's active ingredient includes a group of compounds called valepotriates. Research shows that these compounds attach to the same brain receptors as tranquilizers. Valerian is not one of the best-tasting or best-smelling herbs, so herbalists recommend that you take one or two 400-milligram capsules (rather than tea or tincture) about 30 minutes before bed for best results.

Lemon balm. For a safe sedative that also soothes your stomach, herbalists suggest a

A Sleeper's Tea

The next time insomnia strikes, try an herbal tea made of chamomile, passionflower, and lemon balm. All three are very mild sedatives.

In a small muslin bag or stainless steel tea ball, combine 1 teaspoon each of the three herbs. Add to a cup of boiling water and steep for a few minutes. Drink a cup of tea at bedtime or whenever you'd like to relax.

When to See the Doctor

Is your forgetfulness due to something serious, such as Alzheimer's disease? The fact that you're worried probably means that you're okay. In general, people whose memory is affected by serious medical conditions usually aren't aware of the problem themselves. "The real danger is not when you're worried, but when other people are worried about you," says Jay Lombard, M.D., assistant clinical professor of neurology at Cornell University Medical Center in New York City.

Still, it's okay to take your memory problems to your doctor, and you definitely should if the problems:

• Have noticeably worsened over the course of a year or less.
• Are accompanied by significant changes in mood or perception.
• Have to do with geographical or spatial orientation.
• Interfere with your day-to-day functioning.

cup of lemon balm tea at bedtime. Chemicals in the plant, called terpenes, help provide a sedative action. Use 1 to 3 teaspoons of the dried herb per cup of just-boiled water. Cover, steep for 10 minutes, and strain.

Chamomile. Chamomile is another herb that has a mild sedative effect. To fall asleep easier, drink a cup or two of chamomile tea before going to bed.

‖ Memory Problems

Let's face it: As we get older—and busier— we tend to lose certain details. It's normal, but it's bothersome and sometimes worrisome. Stress and fatigue can cause not only memory lapses but also, if they continue too long, other health problems. Once you've accounted for

(and corrected) external factors that may be blunting your thinking, sharpen your memory and concentration further with these herbal helpers.

Ginkgo. Improve blood flow to your brain and enhance your brain's ability to use oxygen by taking 120 to 240 milligrams of ginkgo a day, divided into two doses. Dozens of studies in Germany and France have substantiated that ginkgo is an excellent herb for improving memory, especially for seniors. Be sure to select ginkgo tablets that are standardized to contain 24 percent ginkgo flavone glycosides and 6 percent terpene lactones—two of ginkgo's most important active ingredients.

Rosemary. For minor concentration lapses and forgetfulness, sniff the scent of rosemary essential oil. Just apply 1 to 3 drops to a tissue, tuck it in your pocket or purse, and inhale as needed. This herb's ability to improve memory and concentration dates back centuries.

Like rosemary, basil is thought to be a great brain booster. To make your own basil memory jar, stuff three or four cotton balls into a 1-ounce glass jar with a lid. Using a dropper, put 3 to 5 drops of basil essential oil into the jar, spreading the drops among the cotton balls. Screw the lid tightly onto the jar. When you need a memory or an alertness boost, open the jar and sniff the scent. Be sure to close the lid tightly, or the essential oil will dry out. Replace when the smell becomes faint.

Menstrual Cramps and Bloating

Womanhood is a wonderful thing, but it has its drawbacks, among them, menstrual cramps and bloating. Cramps are the result of a release of hormones called prostaglandins that cause uterine blood vessels to tighten, reducing blood flow. This makes the uterine muscle flex in what you feel as a painful cramp. As for bloating, blame it on a drop in the female hormone progesterone in the 7 to 10 days before your menstrual cycle. Depletion of progesterone causes salt and water retention throughout your body.

The following herbal remedies may help regulate hormones so that cramping and bloating become less severe.

Cramp bark and valerian. If you have intense cramps and need relief right now, herbalists suggest blending 3 teaspoons of cramp bark tincture and 5 teaspoons of valerian tincture.

Add ½ to 3½ teaspoons of this mixture to a small amount of warm water and drink as needed. Cramp bark relaxes muscles and soothes painful spasms. Valerian contains compounds that relieve muscle spasms and curb anxiety.

Black haw. This herb contains an aspirin-like compound that lessens the pain. Make a tea by adding 2 teaspoons of dried black haw per cup of water. Boil for 10 minutes, cool, strain, and drink up to 3 cups a day. If you tend to get severe cramps, herbalists recommend that you start taking this tea a few days before you expect your period—don't wait until the pain becomes overwhelming.

Dandelion. The leaves of this familiar weed act as a potent diuretic that can effectively reduce uncomfortable bloating and swelling before and during menstruation. Take two capsules twice a day.

Dried dandelion can also be used as part of a hormone-balancing tea that can help prevent menstrual cramps. To make the tea, combine one-quarter part dried chasteberry with one part each of dried wild yam, ginger, and yellow dock. Add two parts each of dried dandelion root, burdock, licorice, and sassafras. Brew the tea by adding 6 tablespoons of the blend to a quart of cold water in a pot. Simmer slowly for 20 minutes, then strain. Drink three to four cups daily for 3 weeks during each menstrual cycle, then stop while you menstruate.

Osteoporosis

Osteoporosis leaves bones weak, brittle, and porous. It may show no outward symptoms for years—which explains why more than 25 million Americans don't even know they have osteoporosis until they sustain a fracture. Women are at particular risk after menopause because production of the female hormone estrogen sharply declines. Estrogen helps bones absorb and retain calcium.

Bone loss actually starts much earlier in a woman's life. After age 35, she'll lose a little every year. In 20 years, she'll be down by 10 to 20 percent. You can slow that loss down, or even add some bone, with regular exercise, calcium supplements, and herbs.

Gentian. Ensure that calcium is properly absorbed from food and vitamin supplements by taking one capsule of gentian root before each meal (a typical capsule is 550 milligrams). This herb prompts stomach acids to effectively break down calcium so that it can be absorbed more completely.

Horsetail. This herb is among the richest plant sources of silicon, a mineral that helps prevent osteoporosis and can be used to treat bone fractures. Natural healers often recommend taking up to nine 350-milligram capsules of horsetail per day, but consult with your herbalist or holistic physician to find the proper dose for you.

You can also take horsetail in tea form by adding about 1 tablespoon of dried horsetail and 1 teaspoon of sugar to each cup of water you use. (The sugar pulls more silicon from the herb.)

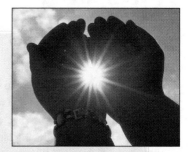

Sunshine Alert

Everybody's watching their exposure to direct sunlight these days, which is good, but there's a downside: a deficiency in vitamin D, the sunshine vitamin, which could be raising your risk of osteoporosis.

A recent study found that out of 290 people between the ages of 18 and 95 admitted to a Boston hospital, 57 percent had vitamin D blood levels low enough to be called deficient. Even more surprising: 46 percent of those who took a daily multivitamin were still deficient, even though most multis contain the recommended Daily Value (DV) for vitamin D (400 international units, or IU).

What to do? Keep taking a multi to get those daily 400 IU, then (if you don't get much direct sunlight), take a calcium supplement with vitamin D. Aim for a daily total of 600 to 800 IU. Milk, nutritional and diet drinks and bars, and fatty canned fish (salmon, mackerel, sardines, herring, and tuna) are also sources of vitamin D.

Bring to a boil in a pan, then simmer for about 3 hours. Strain the leaves. Allow the tea to cool before drinking.

Nettle, oatstraw, and red clover. These herbs are rich in minerals that can help keep bones strong. To get their best medicinal properties, make herbal infusions—stronger than tea—by brewing a batch overnight. Drink over the next day or two.

Premenstrual Syndrome

What we call premenstrual syndrome, or PMS, can manifest itself with more than 150 possible symptoms, so it isn't a simple condition to relieve. For that reason herbalists working with individual women tend to create customized PMS formulas which match their specific needs. Generally, they choose herbs that, when used over a period of months, help balance hormones, stop mood swings, and improve liver function, which helps your body to eliminate excess hormones more effectively. Here are three herbs to try.

Chasteberry. Herbal experts say that chasteberry seems to work by elevating levels of progesterone, the female hormone that rules the second half of the menstrual cycle. To make a tea, use 1 teaspoon of the dried herb per cup of boiling water. Steep for 20 minutes, strain, then drink up to three cups per day.

Yarrow. When PMS causes your abdomen to swell, reverse bloating with yarrow, herbal healers suggest. Combine one-half part dried yarrow and one part dried chasteberry to make a tea. Then use 1 teaspoon of this mix per

Calcium Booster

Mood swings and depression of PMS got you down? Try calcium. When 466 women with PMS took 1,200 milligrams of calcium (as calcium carbonate) every day for 3 months, their psychological symptoms were reduced by 45 percent.

cup of boiling water. Steep for 20 minutes, strain, and sip up to three cups daily. A mild diuretic, yarrow also stimulates the liver, which helps balance hormones.

Passionflower. This herb can help ease anxiety and calm nervous tension, two characteristic symptoms of PMS. Use the dried aerial parts of the herb—the vine, stem, or leaf—in either a tea or as a tincture.

Prostate Problems

More than half the men in the United States over age 50 have problems related to swollen prostates, a condition known as benign prostatic hyperplasia, or BPH. The prostate is a walnut-size gland that produces the fluid that carries sperm. The problem with an enlarged prostate is the gland's location: It encircles the urethra (the tube that carries urine from the bladder) like an inflatable life preserver. An overinflated prostate constricts the urethra, causing discomfort and urinary problems.

BPH is not cancer and does not increase your chances of developing prostate cancer. Doctors aren't sure exactly what causes it. Nonetheless, any man with symptoms of BPH should go to a doctor and undergo a couple of tests—a digital rectal exam of the prostate and a blood test—to make sure that prostate cancer isn't the culprit behind his frequent trips to the bathroom. The American Cancer Society urges all men to get these tests once a year from the time they are 50 years old, or sooner (around age 45) if they have a family history of prostate cancer.

If your doctor determines that you have BPH, there are several herbs that can help.

Saw palmetto. Nearly a dozen studies have shown that saw palmetto, which comes from the berry of a dwarf palm tree that grows in the southeastern United States and the Caribbean, is effective in the treatment of BPH. Take 160 milligrams twice daily of the standardized extract in capsule form. Look for brands that say they provide 85 to 95 percent of fatty acids and sterols. Take this dose until symptoms improve, then lower the dose to the lowest possible to keep symptoms under control.

Pygeum. Elevated cholesterol levels within the prostate gland are associated with BPH, and this herb can help lower them. It also works to decrease inflammation. Make sure that you choose a product that is standardized to 13 percent total sterols. Take 100 milligrams twice a day of standardized extract in capsule form. Take

NATURALFACT

If you have to urinate frequently because of prostate problems, try limiting your use of antihistamines and over the counter cold remedies. Both can increase the amount of pressure the bladder puts on the prostate.

pygeum at this dose until symptoms improve, then lower the dose to the lowest possible to keep symptoms under control.

Nettle. The active ingredients in this herb suppress prostatic cell growth and also decrease inflammation. Take 120 milligrams twice daily of a standardized extract in capsule form until symptoms improve, then lower the dose to the lowest possible to keep symptoms under control.

‖ Psoriasis

Psoriasis is a skin condition caused by super-fast skin growth. In the normal sequence of skin creation, it takes about a month for skin to grow, mature, and fall off. But when you have psoriasis, that process is accelerated. New skin can come and go in as little as 3 days. Since your body can't get rid of new skin that quickly, you end up with too much inventory, in the form of white, crusty lesions that usually develop on fast-growth areas like the elbows, knees, scalp, chest, and back.

Since there is no known cure for psoriasis, herbal treatments are mainly useful for soothing the skin and quelling the itching. See your doctor if the psoriasis does not respond to these remedies.

Flaxseed oil. Flaxseed oil has been shown to improve a number of skin conditions, including psoriasis. Add a daily tablespoon of the oil to food or juice.

Goldenseal. Goldenseal contains substances that stop your body from creating polyamines, chemicals that are linked to psoriasis. Take 200 milligrams of the herb for 2 weeks, three times a day, then reduce to once a day for a month. Stop taking it if you experience no results after 6 weeks.

Chamomile cream. Chamomile cream is an anti-inflammatory agent that helps soothe dry, flaky skin. Rub it on as often as you like, and continue using until your skin clears up.

‖ Sore Throat

Like a magnet, the throat attracts viruses and other airborne irritants that cling to its delicate tissues. Usually, your body finds a way to quickly eradicate the irritant, and you are never consciously aware that it existed. But when conditions are right, the invader settles in and reproduces in your throat. Other mischief makers are smoking, dry air, environmental pollution, bacterial infections, and stomach acid reflux.

You should always see a doctor if your sore throat is accompanied by a rash, earache, discolored mucus, pus-covered tonsils, a high temperature (over 100°F), chest pain, or shortness of breath. Otherwise, you can pretty much treat your sore throat on your own. If you have a cold or flu, check out the remedies for those maladies as well (see "Colds" on page 113 and "Flu" on page 122). In the meantime, try these herbs.

Echinacea. This is the top herbal remedy for stimulating the immune system, and it can be useful in combating sore throat in two ways. Gargling with water and echinacea tincture will put your sore throat on the mend sooner rather than later. Use warm water and

It's Grape for the Skin

Oregon grape is attracting attention in England as a treatment for psoriasis and eczema.

No double-blind studies exist to prove that Oregon grape helps skin problems, but Douglas Schar, a London-based herbalist, is in the process of conducting his own trials, and the results look promising. Why? Schar has a theory. "The herb contains berberine," he says, "which we know constricts capillaries. In inflammatory skin conditions, capillaries dilate and fluids seep into surrounding tissues. Oregon grape seems to reduce the tendency toward inflammation."

The key to success with Oregon grape is long-term use, says Schar—3 months minimum and up to a year for lasting results. Either take 1½ teaspoons twice a day in tincture form or drink ½ cup of Oregon grape root tea twice a day. Prepare the tea by boiling 2 teaspoons of Oregon grape root bark in 4 ounces of water for 5 minutes. Strain and sip.

Tea Time

When it comes to soothing sore throats, it's hard to beat a cup of hot tea with lemon and honey. In addition to the psychological benefits, it's the hot water that's actually doing most of the work, says ear, nose, and throat specialist Toni M. Levine, M.D., assistant professor of otolaryngology at Northwestern University in Chicago. It relieves inflammation and washes away nasal drainage that irritates the back of the throat. Inhaling the steam also helps loosen up congestion.

The basic recipe couldn't be simpler: Brew a cup of your favorite hot tea, squeeze in a wedge of lemon or a little concentrated lemon juice, and stir in 1 to 2 teaspoons of honey. Let it cool for a few minutes before sipping. Repeat as needed.

add 40 drops of echinacea. In the meantime, taking 200 milligrams of echinacea in capsule form four times a day for up to 5 days will help give your body the strength that it needs to roust your infection.

Two other herbal immune system stimulants are astragalus and goldenseal. As with the echinacea, take 200 milligrams in capsule form four times a day for up to 5 days.

Sage and eucalyptus. Combined in a tea, these herbs have anti-inflammatory and antibacterial properties that will heal and soothe simultaneously. Steep 2 teaspoons of dried sage and eucalyptus leaves in 8 ounces of boiling water for 20 to 30 minutes. Let the tea cool, then gargle with it throughout the day as needed.

Rose hips. This herb is loaded with vitamin C that will be quickly absorbed when ingested as a tea. Place 2 tablespoons of rose hips into a nonaluminum pot. Add a cup of water. Cover the pot tightly. Let simmer for 20 to 30 minutes. Strain the tea into a cup with a coffee filter and add freshly squeezed lemon juice and honey to taste.

Urinary Tract Infections

If you have a frequent, urgent need to urinate accompanied by a burning sensation or strong-smelling or cloudy urine, you may have a urinary tract infection (UTI). Women get these far more frequently than men, in part because woman are anatomically more vulnerable to bacterial invasion than men are (their urethras are shorter, making it easier for bacteria to reach the bladder), and in part because things like diaphragms, douches, and spermicides can help set the stage for infection.

Herbs can help prevent UTIs when they're teamed with good hygiene and healthy habits. Wipe from front to back after you go to the toilet to keep bacteria away from the urethra. Drink up to eight glasses of filtered water a day to speed bacteria-infected urine on its way. And go when you feel the urge; holding it in allows bacteria to flourish.

If you've had UTIs in the past and your doctor has ruled out kidney problems, you might want to try herbal remedies for a few days. After that, visit your doctor because some antibiotics may be in order. Also be sure to see a doctor if you have blood in your urine, chills, nausea, vomiting, or lower back pain.

Cranberry. This is an old folk remedy for UTIs that really works. Research has shown that a substance in cranberry keeps infection-causing bacteria from sticking to the lining of the bladder and urethra.

Cranberry can be consumed in a variety of forms. One option is drinking 8 ounces of cranberry juice a day until the symptoms subside. Capsules are more convenient and are even safe for pregnant women. Take two or three capsules containing at least 400 milligrams each of cranberry extract every day until the infection clears up. A third option is cranberry tea. Fill a tea ball with dried cranberries, place the ball in a cup of boiling water, steep for 20 minutes, and drink. Consume three to four cups a day during an infection.

Parsley. This common herb turns out to be an excellent diuretic. To make a tea, pour a cup of boiling water over a few sprigs of crushed fresh parsley or 1 teaspoon of dried parsley. Let the herb steep for 5 to 10 minutes, then strain and drink. Consume one cup two or three times a day until the infection clears up.

‖ Warts

Warts, which are actually benign skin tumors, are caused by a family of viruses called human papillomavirus (HPV). A suppressed immune system seems to increase a woman's susceptibility to them.

Getting rid of warts doesn't always eliminate the virus that caused them in the first place, so natural healers suggest a two-pronged strategy for achieving a lasting solution: Bolster your immune system so that it can better battle viruses, and use

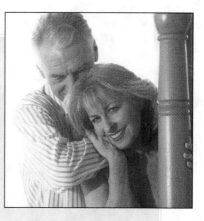

The Love Bug

If you've experienced a recent surge of urinary tract infections (UTIs), Viagra could be—indirectly—the culprit. One group of doctors in Georgia noticed a rise in UTI complaints among women patients between the ages of 55 and 75. "We checked our records and found that every one of their spouses had been given a prescription for Viagra," says Henry Patton, M.D., one of the doctors. Sexual activity can lead to UTIs because rubbing in the genital area can introduce bacteria into the woman's urethra. Clearly, the women were having more fun in bed, but increasing their chances of infection in the process.

herbs that work on the surface to shrink these little growths.

Birch bark. People all over the world have relied on this herb for centuries. It contains two antiviral compounds, betulin and betulinic acid, in addition to salicylates, which are approved by the FDA to treat warts.

If you have access to fresh birch bark, tape a piece of moistened bark, with the inner side down, directly to the wart. If you can't get your hands on some bark, brew some birch bark tea by adding a teaspoon or two of powdered bark to a cup of boiling water. Steep for 10 minutes. You can drink it as a tea or rub it directly on the wart.

Echinacea. Fortify your immune system so that it can defeat wart viruses by taking two 250-milligram capsules of echinacea twice per day.

Basil. This aromatic herb contains many antiviral compounds that have the potential to make warts disappear. Simply pack the crushed leaves over the wart and cover with a bandage. Apply fresh basil daily for 5 to 7 days.

Chapter 12

An Herbal Guide to Menopause

A natural part of life, not an illness; here's how to smooth the transition

For a good part of this century, menopause was thought of almost as a disease, an event to be dreaded before it happened and mourned when it did. That view, happy to say, can be considered obsolete.

Among herbalists—and many women—menopause is viewed with an attitude of acceptance and sometimes even anticipation. "Menopause is not a disorder—it's a powerful and exciting transition," says Rosemary Gladstar, director of the Sage Mountain herbal education center in East Barre, Vermont, and author of *Herbal Healing for Women.* "As long as a woman takes really good care of herself and uses natural support, menopause doesn't have to be the trauma that so many of us fear."

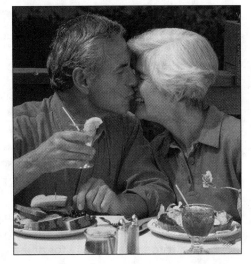

Handle the Challenges

Of course, menopause does have its challenges, hot flashes, changes in periods, and seesawing moods among them. Suddenly, it seems, the body you've known so well for four to five decades just isn't behaving as it once did. Herbs can help.

We interviewed some of the country's top woman herbalists for their recommendations on how to treat menopause problems the natural way. Here's what they said.

Hot Flashes

We don't really know what causes hot flashes—not surprisingly, the body's reactions to hormone changes are suspected—but we do know that as many as 65 to 80 percent of women will experience them at some point during their transitions to menopause. We also know they're unpredictable and uncomfortable. The following herbs can help you put the chill on.

Black cohosh and motherwort. Black cohosh helps normalize hormone fluctuations prior to menopause, says Patricia Howell, a professional member of the American Herbalists Guild and director of the Living with Herbs Institute in Atlanta. She recommends mixing two parts of motherwort tincture with one part black cohosh tincture.

Start with ¼ teaspoon of the formula, mixed into a small amount of water or a cup of tea, three times a day. Some herbalists recommend increasing the dosage to ½ teaspoon three times a day, but that dosage may cause nausea, says Howell.

If that happens, take it less often.

Motherwort has traditionally been used to lower blood pressure (a use modern research has since verified as effective), which may be why it's considered a help for hot flashes. Motherwort also has sedative qualities to ease the insomnia

Taming the Volcanic Hot Flash

For some women, menopause follows surgical removal of the ovaries or chemotherapy or radiation treatments that can destroy the ovaries, says Susun S. Weed, an herbalist and herbal educator from Woodstock, New York, and author of *Menopausal Years: The Wise Woman's Way.* For them, hot flashes may be especially frequent and intense. "Volcanic hot flashes are to a normal hot flash as a tidal wave is to a normal wave," she says.

Twenty-five to 30 drops of motherwort tincture can stem the tide, Weed says. And for the long term, she recommends 30 to 90 drops of chasteberry tincture three times a day for at least 13 months.

that troubles many menopausal women, notes Gladstar.

Dang gui, chasteberry, and damiana. This trio of herbs is recommended by Andrew Weil, M.D., director of the program in integrative medicine at the at the University of Arizona College of Medicine in Tucson and author of *Spontaneous Healing*. Damiana is a nervous-system tonic, said to ease depression and anxiety. Don't use dang gui while menstruating, spotting, or bleeding heavily, because it can increase blood loss.

Take one dropperful each of the three herbs in tincture form once a day at midday, Dr. Weil says. Continue until your hot flashes cease, then taper off the tinctures gradually.

Night Sweats

Hot flashes that strike while you're asleep are called night sweats, and sometimes feelings of terror or anxiety will precede them. Here's how to help yourself through them.

Sage. Garden sage is famed for the way it reduces or even eliminates night sweats. It acts fast, within a few hours, and a single cup of infusion can stave off the sweats for up to 2 days, says Susun S. Weed, an herbalist and herbal educator from Woodstock, New York,

NATURALFACT

"Cohosh" is a Native American word that means "knobby rough roots." There are four different cohoshes—red, white, blue, and black, all referring to widely different native plants. Native Americans were the first to use black cohosh for female ailments.

and author of *Menopausal Years: The Wise Woman's Way*. What's more, you probably have a bottle of sage sitting on your spice rack. Just make sure it's still nice and aromatic before you use it medicinally.

To make a sage infusion, put 4 heaping tablespoons of dried sage in a cup of hot water. Cover tightly and steep for 4 hours or more.

Irregular Periods and Flooding

Your cycles used to be regular, but now they're not. You used to know roughly how many tampons or napkins you'd use during each period, but now you haven't a clue. Nothing about your period is as it used to be. Sometimes herbs can even out irregular menses; sometimes they can't. Weed suggests trying these herbal remedies.

Chasteberry. Although it's slow to act, chasteberry tincture is highly recommended for women who are bothered by menopausal irregularities. Weed recommends a dropperful in a small glass of water or juice two or three times a day for 6 to 8 weeks after every irregular period.

Cinnamon. Cinnamon bark invigorates the blood, helps regulate the menstrual cycle, and checks flooding, says Weed. For heavy bleeding, sip a cup of cinnamon infusion or use 5 to 10 drops of tincture once or twice a day, or chew on a cinnamon stick. You can also simply sprinkle cinnamon powder freely on food, advises Weed.

Lady's-mantle. In a clinical study, 5 to 10 drops of lady's-mantle tincture controlled menstrual hemorrhage in virtually all of the 300 women who participated, says Weed. When taken after flooding began, lady's-mantle took 3 to 5 days to become effective. When taken for 1 to 2 weeks before menstruation, it prevented flooding. Weed suggests using 5 to 10 drops of the fresh plant tincture three times a day for up to 2 weeks out of every month.

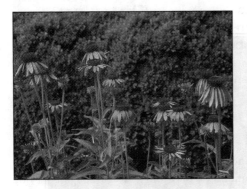

Vaginal Dryness

After menopause, your vaginal lining may begin to thin and dry out because of the lack of estrogen. As a result, having sex may hurt, and you may find yourself with a vexing vaginal infection. Here are some herbal remedies to help keep your love life flowing.

Witch hazel and aloe vera. Try a blend of equal parts of distilled witch hazel and pure aloe vera gel, used as needed as a vaginal lubricant before and during sex, suggests Gladstar. You can also mix it with some slippery elm powder, which makes the liquid even more, well, slippery, she says.

Stem the Tide

When heavy bleeding is a symptom of your premenopausal periods, try to consume more iron from herbs and food sources, recommends Susun S. Weed, an herbalist and herbal educator from Woodstock, New York, and author of *Menopausal Years: The Wise Woman's Way*. You'll feel more energetic and alive within 2 weeks, and your flooding will diminish noticeably by your next period, she adds.

Herbal sources of iron include dandelion leaves, milk thistle seed, dang gui, black cohosh, echinacea, and peppermint, according to Weed. Food sources include leafy greens, tofu, raisins, carrots, beets, pumpkin, tomatoes, cauliflower, mushrooms, soybeans, and salmon. Of course, lean red meat is the best source of iron, because it contains heme iron, which is readily absorbed by the body.

Evening primrose oil. Try massaging your vaginal area, daily or whenever you need some extra lubrication, with primrose oil alone or with a combination of primrose oil and vitamin E oil, suggests Amanda McQuade Crawford, a practicing herbalist in Ojai, California, and author of *Herbal Remedies for Women*. Clary sage essential oil (5 drops per ounce) can be substituted for the primrose if you prefer. Either oil will make your vaginal tissues moister and more supple.

Comfrey. "Comfrey ointment is the ally of choice when skin needs flexible strength," says Weed. Use the ointment to keep vaginal tissues moist, strong, and supple by rubbing it in morning and evening and using it during love play. Your vulva will be noticeably plumper and moister within 3 weeks, Weed promises.

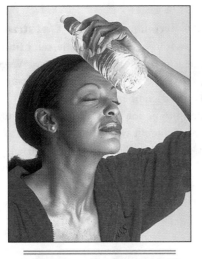

As many as 65 to 80 percent of women will experience hot flashes at some point during their transitions to menopause.

You can also do what French courtesans used to do: Brew up 2 quarts of comfrey leaf infusion, then strain it, rewarm to a comfortable temperature, pour it into a small tub, and "sitz" yourself in it until it cools, says Weed.

Mood Swings

In menopause, you can be merry one moment and maniacal the next, without any rhyme or reason, it seems. These fluctuations may be the result of excess water retention, which can lead to depression and anxiety. Herbs can remedy that situation.

Dandelion tea. Contrary to what you might think, the solution to fluid retention is to drink more fluid, not less, says Gladstar, because water is an absolute necessity for

The Conventional Method

Conventional medicine treats menopause as a deficiency disease of estrogen. Although doctors often prescribe hormone-replacement therapy (HRT), replacement hormones can't fully mimic your body's natural cycle. And some women stop taking HRT after experiencing the side effects, which can include menstrual-like bleeding, bloating, irritability, cramps, headaches, and depression.

correcting fluid balance. She recommends drinking at least 2 quarts of water or mild diuretic herbal tea, like dandelion or nettle, daily.

Another option is unsweetened cranberry juice, which serves as a refreshing tonic for the kidneys. If it's just too tart for you, dilute it with water and add a bit of honey, Gladstar says. And, if you can't find unsweetened cranberry juice, regular cranberry juice, such as Ocean Spray, is just fine, she adds.

Oatstraw. Drinking oatstraw infusion freely can banish irritability and strengthen the nerves, says Weed.

Skullcap. A skullcap tincture strengthens the nerves, eases oversensitivity, and helps promote deep, sound sleep, says Weed. She uses 4 to 8 drops mornings and evenings when she's feeling "fried, stressed out, wired, or just wound up." (Do not confuse it with Chinese skullcap, though, which has entirely different properties.)

Chapter 13

Sex after Marriage: It's Not a Myth!

How herbs can put the oomph back in your love life

Is sex something that only the young enjoy? Sometimes it seems that way. Certainly, there's nothing romantic about the whole clash and clamor of modern life. Busy schedules don't leave much time for lovemaking. And even if they did, stress acts as a bucket of ice-cold water on sexual desire. Physiological changes can limit the libido, too, for men in particular. *Erectile dysfunction* is a medical term that a lot of frustrated couples are learning about.

None of these sexual problems need be taken lying down. Healthy living in general can keep you and your lover on intimate terms indefinitely, while herbs can play a key supporting role in your sexual longevity prescription. Here are recommendations from some of the country's leading herbalists.

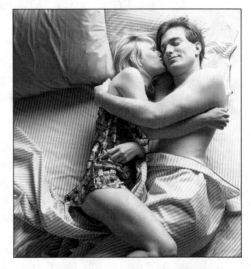

Low Sexual Desire

Remember the last time you actually lusted for someone? When you felt faint with desire? When you tore the clothes off your partner and leaped into bed?

Believe it or not, you can rekindle that kind of passion with the help of the herbal remedies that follow. We'll tell you how in a second, but first, a brief reality check. Lots of physical and psychological issues—everything from recurring vaginal infections to depression—can put the kibosh on your love life, and the following herbal fire starters aren't going to address them. If you've checked out your overall health with your doctor and still yearn for more sexual intimacy, then give botanicals a try. Be aware, however, that libido-enhancing herbs are not recommended for pregnant women.

Sandalwood, rose, or amber. Set the stage for passion by scenting the bedroom (or any room) with a few potent droplets of sandalwood, rose, or amber essential oil, suggests Aviva Romm, a certified professional midwife, herbalist, and professional member of the American Herbalists Guild who practices in Bloomfield Hills, Michigan. "Sandalwood is a traditional aphrodisiac," Romm says. "It makes you feel very centered in your body, very aware of physical sensation. Rose and amber both have long associations with love and sensuality."

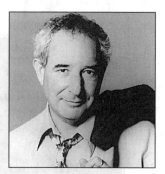

HEALING SPOTLIGHT
Michael Tucker

Actor Michael Tucker, who for 8 successful years played nebbish attorney Stuart Markowitz on the TV series *L.A. Law,* is a seasoned user of alternative medicine. He and his wife, Jill Eickenberry (who starred as Markowitz's wife, Ann Kelsey, on the series), use acupuncture and homeopathy regularly, and Tucker has long practiced meditation.

Tucker's deepest passion, though, may be tantric sex, an ancient Eastern discipline that treats sexual intercourse as a form of spiritual exercise. Tucker believes that making love to his wife "at least twice a day" has had more to do with keeping his cholesterol down than exercising or watching his diet.

"There are times during intimacy when it feels as if Jill and I are in an elevated state of being," he says. "We get high from this. There are a lot of ways to get high, but this is the best I've ever found."

There are several easy ways to "perfume" the air with sensuality. One is to buy a diffuser ring. These devices, available in health food stores or by mail, fit over a standard light bulb. When you place a few drops of essential oil in the ring, the heat from the bulb releases the fragrance. Simpler still, just add a few drops of essential oil to a cup of warm water (the heat will release the aroma) or place 5 drops of essential oil and ½ cup of water in an atomizer, then shake and spray into the air.

The same essential oils, when added to massage oil, bring new sensual dimensions to a full-body massage before lovemaking. "You need only a few drops of essential oil to scent a massage oil," Romm says. "For example, to an ounce of jojoba oil, add a total of 8 or 9 drops of sandalwood, rose, or amber or a combination of them."

Partners can massage each other from head to toe; concentrate first on relaxation by working on tense spots such as the upper back, then let your touch become slower, more caressing, even arousing. Include erogenous zones like the backs of the knees and the inner thighs.

Damiana tea. Damiana has a long reputation in folk medicine as an aphrodisiac. "It seems to lower anxiety and open the door to sensual expression," says Margi Flint, a professional member of the American Herbalists Guild who teaches herbal approaches to health at Tufts University School of Medicine in Boston.

To make a quick damiana tea, steep 1 teaspoon of dried leaves in a cup of boiling water for 10 minutes. Or just use damiana tincture. "If you want to take damiana on a regular basis as a tonic, use 15 to 20 drops of tincture three times a day," Romm notes. "To boost passion for a sexual encounter, try 20 to 30 drops in ¼ cup of warm water, taken about an hour in advance."

NATURALFACT

A man's chances of having erection trouble increase dramatically with age. One study found that men ages 50 to 59 experience difficulties with erections more than three times as often as men ages 18 to 29.

Put a Cork in It

Some herbs are widely believed to boost our sex lives enormously, but probably don't. We're talking about barley, hops, and other herbal beverages that are fermented to produce alcohol.

To raise the blood alcohol level to 0.05, a 150-pound man would have to drink roughly three mixed drinks in 1 to 2 hours. One study found that men who had a blood alcohol level of 0.06 took significantly longer to ejaculate. Not so bad, you say? Consider that men whose blood alcohol level was 0.9—nearly the level of impairment in many states—were unable to ejaculate at all.

Gingerroot. Herbs that stimulate circulation can enhance sexual feelings by increasing blood flow to the genital region. Romm recommends adding 1 tablespoon of grated gingerroot, 7 to 10 cloves, 2 to 3 cinnamon sticks, 4 to 5 black peppercorns, and 7 to 10 cardamom pods to 2 cups of water. Simmer for 20 minutes, strain, and add small amounts of milk and honey to taste. "For a really nice touch, add ¼ teaspoon of vanilla," Romm says. "Vanilla comes from the orchid family, and orchids are incredibly sensual flowers. It's an aphrodisiac."

Tonic herbs. Both men and women can stimulate their sexual energy by using "tonic herbs," which stimulate energy overall. Romm recommends taking daily doses of angelica, dang gui, ginseng,

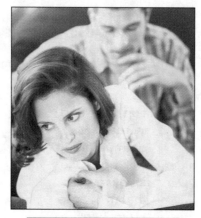

"We must reckon with the possibility that something in the nature of the sexual instinct itself is unfavorable to the realization of complete satisfaction."

—Sigmund Freud

chasteberry, or saw palmetto as tinctures. "Use ½ teaspoon to 1 full teaspoon in ¼ cup of warm water twice a day," she says. "You can take them for 3 months or longer, since tonic herbs can be used safely for longer periods. But give your body a break. For one day a week, don't take the herb, then every 3 weeks, take a week off."

Nourishing herbs. Herbs that strengthen your system in general will help with sexuality and passion, Romm notes. Over time, using herbs such as nettle and red clover will provide a feeling of well-being and emotional stability. Women may also notice more vaginal lubrication. Look for results after about a month, Romm says.

Among her favorite herbs for building and sustaining passion is ashwaganda, a kidney-nour-

Sexual Magic

For centuries, herbalists have whispered of a love potion guaranteed to turn even the limpest lover into a raging volcano of sexual passion. The magic substance bears the exotic name *yohimbe.*

Derived from the bark of an African tree, yohimbe supposedly works by forcing blood to erectile tissues. However, herbalists stress that yohimbe has plenty of problems. Side effects include potentially dangerous elevations in heart rate and blood pressure, anxiety, and hallucinations. Given those risks, yohimbe is one love potion that should be used only under the supervision of a physician.

ishing botanical. "Add about ½ teaspoon of ashwaganda powder to a cup of milk, bring it just to a boil, then sweeten with honey," she says. "You can drink this every day."

Or try shatavari. The Sanskrit name of this Indian herb means "she who possesses 100 husbands," Romm says. "You could combine it with the ashwaganda in milk, using ½ teaspoon to 1 full teaspoon of shatavari." The same amount of shatavari can be mixed with a little honey and eaten as a sweet paste, she adds.

> ## NATURALFACT
>
> In a survey of more than 1,000 American adults, 45 percent of those responding cited stress as the biggest hindrance to sex. Women were more likely to give that response than men.

Erection Problems

Erectile dysfunction is a far more common problem than men want to admit. Researchers speculate that as many as 15 million American men experience it.

The source of the problem can be physical or psychological, or both. The penis is designed to expand and hold blood when it rushes in. If the arteries leading to the penis are clogged, if the valves that hold blood in are leaky, or if the tissue and muscles that usually expand are creaky from disuse, erectile capability will be diminished. Fatigue and depression can also play a role.

The best insurance policies against erectile dysfunction are exercise and a healthy diet. Maintaining a regular sex life helps, too. If there are psychological issues involved, a visit to a coun-selor may be in order. In the meantime, herbs may be able to give you (or your partner) a lift.

Ginkgo. Available at most natural food and supplement stores, gingko increases blood and oxygen flow to the extremities, including the penis. In one study, 60 men with erectile difficulties were given daily ginkgo supplements for a period of 12 to 18 months. After a 6-month period, 50 percent of the men who took the ginkgo reported that they had regained potency.

Ginseng. A traditional Chinese virility tonic, ginseng (the Chinese variety, called panax) has been shown in several studies to boost sexual activity. The effect builds over time, which means that you'll have to take it for a few months before seeing the benefits. Take capsules containing 15 percent of ginsenosides daily.

Muira puama. Also known as potency wood, this herb derived from a Brazilian shrub has a long history as an herbal treatment for impotence, and at least one landmark study showed that it did indeed help a slight majority of men—51 percent of those who took it daily for 2 weeks—improve their erectile function. Take capsules containing 300 milligrams once a day.

Saw palmetto. Best known as a treatment for prostate troubles, saw palmetto can also have a positive impact on erections. The reason? An enlarged prostate can impair bloodflow, interfering with sexual performance. Take two capsules containing 160 milligrams each daily.

NATURAL HEALING THROUGH HISTORY

Trotula of Salerno: A Woman of Distinction

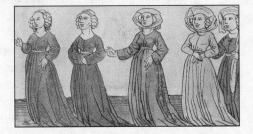

The history of herbal healing is in many respects a feminine history. Men may have brought home the bacon, but women tended the gardens and provided the green medicine.

Often, these services went unrecorded, and so, uncredited. An exception was Trotula of Salerno, an eleventh-century herbalist and midwife who has been called the first woman professor of medicine.

Trotula was a member of a noble Italian family in Salerno, Italy. Salerno was known in the Middle Ages as a great center of healing. People flocked there for its climate, its mineral springs, its hospitals, and its doctors. The city was also home of one of the premiere medical schools in Europe— the only such school to admit women. It's believed that Trotula not only graduated but became chair of the medicine department there as well. She is also said to have maintained an extensive clinical practice and to have written medical textbooks that were studied for hundreds of years.

Trotula was especially well-known for her work in obstetrics and gynecology, and herbs played a prominent role in her ministrations. A distressed mother in labor, for example, might be bathed in a warm bath laced with chickpeas, flaxseed, barley, and cooked mallow, then gently massaged with oil of violets or oil of roses. After the birth, if the woman's breasts were painful from nursing, she might be encouraged to soothe them with a poultice of potter's earth blended with vinegar. Trotula was one of the first medical practitioners to suggest that infertility might be a problem originating with the husband as well as the wife—"radical thinking indeed in eleventh-century Italy," writes historian Elisabeth Brooke.

It is true that Trotula's writings are laden with superstition and magic, but they also display the observations and insights of a keen scientific mind. So advanced were Trotula's writings, in fact, that many historians question whether she has been given credit for work actually produced by a man. More contemporary female historians have not been as skeptical on this score.

Evidence that Trotula was a highly honored woman can be gathered from attendance at her funeral: The line of mourners was said to stretch 2 miles long. The great healer's reputation also earned her a place in literary history. She is said to have been the model for the midwife in Geoffrey Chaucer's *The Canterbury Tales*.

Chapter 14

Herbs Plus Drugs Can Equal Trouble

Taking both can have unexpected consequences; here's what to watch out for

You're taking prescription medications, but you'd also like to use herbs. Is that a problem?

That's the most frequent question posed to one of the world's top herb experts, Varro E. Tyler, Ph.D., Sc.D., distinguished professor emeritus of pharmacognosy and dean emeritus of Purdue University School of Pharmacy and Pharmacal Sciences in West Lafayette, Indiana, and author of *The Honest Herbal*.

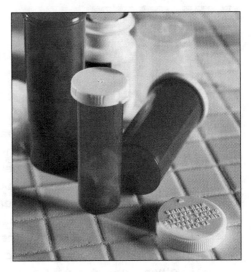

There are no easy answers. In America, herbs are sold as dietary supplements, not as drugs. As a result, herbs aren't tested for safety as rigorously as drugs are, and neither are potentially harmful drug-herb interactions.

Still, with our growing experience with herb use, we now recognize some of the potential dangers.

Antidepressants

Since it became renowned as the herb for the blues, St. John's wort has become one of the hottest-selling herbal supplements. It's not yet known, however, how safe it might be to combine St. John's wort with prescription antidepressants such as Tofranil and Prozac. That's because experts don't really know how this herb works.

Here's Dr. Tyler's advice: Don't take St. John's wort with any antidepressant drug unless such a combination is recommended by your doctor. He adds another, special caution: Never take the herb ephedra (also known as ma huang) with antidepressants like phenelzine (Nardil). These drugs are known as monoamine oxidase (MAO) inhibitors, and ephedra can cause serious toxic reactions ranging from liver damage to severe high blood pressure if combined with MAO inhibitors. In fact, avoid ephedra altogether unless you're under the care of a practitioner experienced in herbs.

Anticoagulants (Blood Thinners)

Some of our most popular herbs lengthen the time that it takes for blood to clot, usually by hindering the ability of blood platelets to clump together. In most cases, this is a good thing. When a clot forms in the brain, it can trigger a stroke. If it occurs in the cardiac arteries, it can cause a heart attack.

Herbs with clot-protective benefits include garlic, ginkgo, ginger, and feverfew. So if you take so-called anticoagulant (anti-clotting) drugs, whether it's over-the-counter aspirin or the potent prescription drug warfarin (Coumadin), use these herbs only after checking with your doctor, Dr. Tyler says.

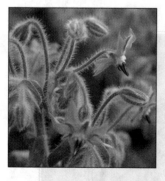

A Slower Pace

We're used to feeling an almost instant effect when we take prescription or over-the-counter drugs. The impact of herbs is usually much more gentle, so much so that you may not notice at first that they're working. The same applies to herbal side effects.

It may help to take notes on your condition after you start taking herbal supplements, suggests Steven Dentali, Ph.D., a natural products chemist with Dentali Associates in Troutdale, Oregon, and a member of the advisory board of the American Botanical Council. That way, the cause-and-effect relationship between the supplement and the disappearance of symptoms, or the appearance of other symptoms, will become clear.

If you're scheduled for surgery, your surgeon will usually tell you to stop taking anticoagulant drugs a few days before the procedure, but you may not be asked about anticoagulant herbs you may be taking. If not, take it upon yourself to ask your doctor. As a matter of fact, it's always a good practice to discuss everything you take—drugs, herbs, or other dietary supplements—with your doctor.

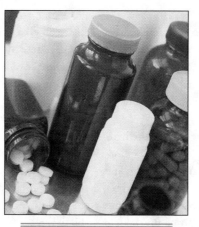

"Just because herbs are readily available or advertised as so-called natural products does not mean that they are completely safe and free of side effects. You really should treat herbs like drugs. They shouldn't be used indiscriminately or taken for fun."

—Eran Ben-Arye, M.D., natural medicine research unit, Hadassah University Hospital in Jerusalem

‖ Diuretics

Herbal stimulant laxatives and diuretics can potentially cause potassium loss, especially if the herbs are used to excess over prolonged periods. When used properly by themselves, none of these herbs pose a serious problem. However, if you use them with the popular diuretic drugs known as thiazide diuretics, you could be headed for trouble.

Thiazide diuretics are common high blood pressure medications, and they're also used to treat the edema (swelling from fluid buildup) that's associated with congestive heart failure. These drugs include Diuril, Saluron, HydroDIURIL, and Naturetin. These drugs can also cause potassium loss, which, if not corrected, can lead to hypokalemia, a serious condition with symptoms that include confusion, muscular weakness, and irregular heartbeat. In some cases, it can even cause you to stop breathing.

Herbs that can potentially drain potassium from your system are stimulant laxatives such as aloe, cascara sagrada, and senna. Licorice can also contribute to potassium loss. Though it takes relatively large doses over long periods of time to cause serious problems, it's probably best not to take licorice either when you take thiazide diuretics.

One good way to avoid potassium loss is to eat foods high in potassium: legumes such as kidney beans, low-fat or fat-free milk, and fruits and vegetables. Each of the following foods contains about 0.5 gram of potassium: 1 cup prune or orange juice, 1 banana, 1 white potato, 7 prunes, 4 figs.

‖ Sedatives (Sleep Aids)

Herbs that sedate or tranquilize, such as kava and valerian, are liable to enhance the effects of drugs that also sedate or tranquilize. Potentially, this could result in dangerous problems—prolonged drowsiness, loss of coordination, or trouble driving or operating machinery. Fortunately, some of the older drugs most likely to produce these sedative effects are rarely prescribed these days. These include secobarbital (Seconal) and phenobarbital (Barbita).

In the place of those heavy hitters, the benzodiazepines such as diazepam (Valium), chlordiazepoxide (Librium), triazolam (Halcion), and flurazepam (Dalmane) are more commonly prescribed today. However, these may also cause problems with selected herbs. To be on the safe side, Dr. Tyler recommends against taking kava or valerian with any sedative or tranquilizing drug.

‖ **Miscellaneous**

Other, usually minor, interactions can occur between herbs and drugs. For example, herbs containing large amounts of mucilage (a gelatinous substance) may slow the absorption of any drug that you take orally if you take them at the same time. These herbs include aloe gel, flaxseed, marshmallow root, and slippery elm bark. To avoid any absorption problem, take the herb and the drug at least several hours apart.

Hundreds of medicinal plants have been shown to lower blood sugar levels in test animals. Some of the better-known ones include bitter melon, cornsilk, dandelion, and prickly pear. When combined with insulin, their effects could result in hypoglycemia. However, such a possibility is relatively rare in this country, where most people with diabetes constantly monitor their blood sugar levels and make the necessary adjustments in the dosage of the antidiabetic drug they're using.

It's likely that other interactions will be discovered in the future as we gain experience using medicinal herbs. In the meantime, it's worth saying again: Consult a qualified medical practitioner (one who has clinical herbal experience) if you have any doubt about the compatibility of herbs and the drugs you take.

NATURAL HEALING IN THE FUTURE

Tracking an Herbal Explosion

Mark Blumenthal is the founder and director of the American Botanical Council, editor of the journal *HerbalGram*, and senior editor of the English translation of Germany's definitive "Commission E" reports on herbal remedies. Here he talks about

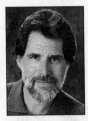 the remarkable growth that herbal medicine has experienced in America over the past decade, and what to expect in the next decade.

Q: What changes have you witnessed in herbal medicine over the past 10 years?

A: Herbal medicine has grown exponentially. For decades in this country, herbs had been discounted as witchcraft, hippie dippie, or folk medicine that many of us never thought doctors would ever take seriously. Today, they're sold in department stores, major drugstore chains have their own generic brands, and major pharmaceutical companies are promoting their own line of herbal products. Herbs have become a major part of the American culture again. They're reclaiming their rightful place.

Q: How are people's attitudes toward herbs today different from 10 years ago?

A: I think that consumer attitudes are more functionally oriented today. In the past, people were more interested in products they wanted to avoid—avoid

sugar, avoid fat, avoid preservatives. Now, people are motivated by a more proactive desire to benefit from herbs. Like ginkgo to enhance memory, St. John's wort for mood elevation, echinacea to help treat symptoms of a cold. People are more aware of medical conditions than ever before and which herbs may help those conditions.

Q: What's the future of herbal medicine?

A: Herbs are here to stay. More and more research will be funded by U.S. herb manufacturers and the U.S. government. This research will generate more articles in the professional and lay press, for example, on the safety and efficacy of St. John's wort versus Prozac for mild to moderate depression, and this will drive sales.

Q: What do you think should happen 10 years from now that isn't happening today?

A: Physicians should consider using botanical medicines instead of conventional drugs in their clinical practice when it is clinically appropriate. These products are effective and, in some cases, such as with saw palmetto and St. John's wort, safer than their prescription drug counterparts. They're also less expensive. The second thing that should happen is that medical schools should and must include botanical medicine in their curriculum because that is what the public is using. They cannot ignore that.

Learning the natural rhythms of your own metabolism can turn you into a weight-loss winner.

Part Six

Natural
Weight
Loss

The natural route to getting slim is also the most effective route.

Chapter 15

Why the Best Diet Is No Diet at All

Get off the weight-loss merry-go-round: five reasons that diets don't work

I t's a strange obsession we have, this dieting thing. We can't look at a piece of fried chicken without worrying about what it will do to our thighs, our bellies, our butts. Our mental calorie counters are always turned on. Cake now minus breakfast tomorrow plus working out tomorrow night equals wearing something other than a tent to the party this weekend.

It gets old. Worse, it doesn't work. Half of those who lose weight by cutting calories regain or exceed their pre-diet weight within a year. Long term, the numbers are even more disheartening. "Ninety-five percent of women who lose weight regain it all within 5 years," says Sue Cummings, R.D., a clinical dietitian at Massachusetts General Hospital in Boston.

There *is* a better way.

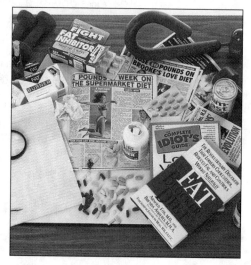

Why Diets Fail

Losing weight is a skill you can learn. The first step is to know what you've been doing wrong up till now. Researchers have spent a lot of time and money studying that question. These are the basic reasons, they say, that we have been dieting like crazy and still gaining weight.

Diets make your fat cells fatter. The fat cells we have in our bodies can grow in size and in number. Every woman, for example, has about 30 billion fat cells, but that number can be increased to 100 billion or so. Diets only speed this fattening process. "Diets act essentially as fitness programs for fat cells," says Debra Waterhouse, R.D., a San Francisco nutritionist and author of _Outsmarting the Female Fat Cell._ "They boost the ability of fat cells to store fat, to take in new fat, and in some cases, to increase their numbers."

Why? Evolution. Fat cells evolved to keep us alive during times of famine, and they react to a low-calorie diet as just that—famine. Fat cells respond to famine, or calorie restriction, by holding on to the fat they already have and by becoming more aggressive at taking in new fat once the diet is over.

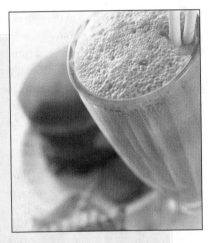

Why Do We Love Fat?

We all know that the double cheeseburger with extra cheese isn't the way to lose weight, but why is it that a million calories have to taste so darn good?

Several reasons. Fat is where the flavor is, for one thing. "Most of the flavor components that we find in foods are fat soluble," says John Erdman, Ph.D., and director of the division of nutritional sciences at the University of Illinois at Urbana-Champaign.

Fat is also a matter of habit, both personal and biological. Our dietary preferences are culturally determined. The French love oil, for example, while Fins are into dairy. Americans lust for cheeseburgers. On a species basis, the fact that fat delivers more calories per bite than other foods means that it was a more efficient foodstuff in the days when dinner had to be chased down and killed. "In our evolutionary history, we didn't have a supermarket around the corner," says Anthony Sclafini, Ph.D., professor of psychology at Brooklyn College of the City University of New York. "So we're programmed to acquire preferences for substances that have a lot of nutrient value."

Diets mess with your enzymes. Our cells manufacture enzymes, tiny protein molecules that, depending on the type, encourage the body to either burn fat or store fat. Dieting can double the number of fat-storing enzymes and halve the number of fat-burning enzymes.

Diets put the brakes on your metabolism. When you diet, you risk starving your body of vital nutrients, because nutrient intake is tied to calorie intake. Very low calorie diets can trigger a complex chain of reactions that will eventually tell your metabolism to stop burning so many calories. You may lose weight initially after cutting calories. Eventually, however, the pounds become harder to drop. Then, when you start eating normally, it takes your metabolic rate a while to get back up to speed—and you gain weight.

Diets make you rebellious. The more you focus on what foods you are allowed to eat and what foods you are not allowed to eat, the more deprived you feel, says Susan Olson, Ph.D., a clinical psychologist and weight-management consultant in Seattle and author of

NATURALFACT

Even if you eat only low-fat foods, portion size matters. Remember, elephants eat nothing but salad, and without the dressing.

Keeping It Off: Winning at Weight Loss. Then you rebel. Instead of just eating a small amount of the "bad" food, you binge, eating well beyond fullness.

"If you say you are going on a diet tomorrow, then you are probably going to stuff yourself tonight," says Dr. Olson. Such binge eating can actually make you wolf down more food than you normally would without the diet.

Binge eating also makes you store more fat than you normally would had you spread the same number of calories throughout the day. "If you eat more calories than your body can burn in a few hours, the remainder will be stored as fat," says Waterhouse.

Diets don't last. You need to change your eating and exercise habits for a lifetime to lose weight and keep it off. By definition, however, diets mean temporary deprivation. So while you may lose a few pounds, once you return to your normal eating habits, the weight returns.

And that, in a nutshell, is the problem. The question is, what can you do about it?

The answer: Plenty.

Chapter 16

47 Weight-Loss Tips That *Do* Work

Guaranteed weight-loss techniques from the real experts—people who used them

O kay. Old-fashioned diets don't work. What does work? We went to the real weight-loss experts—regular folks—to get their tips for taking it off and keeping it off.

What interested us most was finding people who had not only lost lots of weight—more than 30 pounds—but who had also found a way to keep the weight off for more than a year. And, of course, we looked

for people who had lost weight naturally: no drugs, no surgery, no crazy, unhealthy diets.

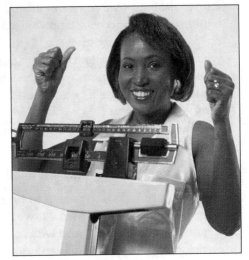

We talked to more than two dozen weight-loss veterans to find out the secrets of their success. Not surprisingly, they changed their eating habits and increased their activity levels. But haven't we all tried that? Why did it work for them and not others? Here is their advice.

Overcome Inertia

The tough part with exercise is getting out there and doing it. Here are the tips that our everyday experts recommend to get you going.

1. Prioritize. The beds may not get made, but Amy, 36, still makes time for exercise. That's how she's kept off more than 80 pounds for 13 years. "I have to schedule it in and let go of other things—like a perfectly clean house," she says.

2. Find a passion. "I have a dance background, and when I found jazzercise, I said, 'Thank God.' If somebody had told me I had to go out and run 5 days a week, I'd still weigh 185 pounds," says Anne, 41, who lost 55 pounds and has kept it off for 13 years.

3. Keep an exercise log. It makes you more accountable. Norma from Dallas, who hangs hers on the refrigerator, checks off six workouts a week dutifully. "If I miss 1 day, I make that my day off for the week."

4. Set a goal. Sign up for some fun runs and try to improve your times. "I went from a 5-K to a 4-miler, then a 5-miler, then a 10-K. As I was building miles and speed, I was getting fitter and losing more weight," says Therese, 42, who lost 80 pounds and recently ran a marathon.

5. Get pumped. "It wasn't until I put on more muscle through resistance training that I was able to keep the weight off—almost effortlessly," says Veronica, 37, who went from a size 18 to an 8. The reason? Muscle burns more calories around the clock.

Support Yourself

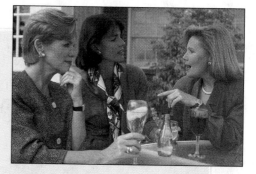

Several of our everyday weight-loss experts mentioned how helpful it was to have a support team in place. One woman had a one-man backup "team" consisting of her fiancé, who was willing to play tennis or ride a bike instead of going out for pizza.

Others found support groups to be helpful. "Hearing someone say she lost 50 pounds would be real motivating," says Therese, 42. "I'd think, 'She's just a normal person like me. If she can lose 50, then I can do it too.'"

Support groups don't have to be professionally organized, either. Debra, 44, started her own. "It was just a bunch of women that got together once a week, and we would compare notes," she says. Not coincidentally, Debra is currently 135 pounds slimmer than she was 13 years ago.

Eat Smart

6. Make changes for the long haul. "I learned how to eat and live with it for the rest of my life," says Barbara, 42, who lost more than 40 pounds and hasn't seen any of them come back in 3 years.

7. Get a grip on reality. "When I started keeping a food diary, I discovered that I was eating somewhere between 3,000 and 4,000 calories a day," says Rebecca, 46, who found the number shocking.

8. Eat mini-meals. Having smaller, more frequent meals can prevent you from getting ravenously hungry and overeating. On average, weight-loss winners eat five times a day.

9. Follow the 90-to-10-percent rule. "If you watch what you eat 90 percent of the time, the other 10 percent is not a problem," says Veronica, who learned this tip from a fitness professional.

10. Eat at the dinner table. If you eat in front of the TV, then every time you nestle in with the remote control, it's a cue to eat. Instead, designate an eating spot for all meals and snacks. "Even when I want potato chips, I set the table just as if I was going to sit down for a full-course meal," says Kathy, 47, who took off more than 100 pounds. "I put a handful of chips on the plate, put the bag away, and then sit down to eat. I never just stand at the counter and eat now."

11. Think before you bite. Creating rituals—such as setting the table like Kathy did or waiting 10 minutes before giving in to a craving—can stop you from eating when you really aren't hungry. "Nine chances out of 10, the chips go back in the cupboard, and I just walk away," says Kathy.

12. Drink up. "Drinking lots of water keeps me from snacking when I'm not hungry, and it gives me more energy," says Therese. "It also stopped what I thought were hunger headaches, which were probably due to dehydration."

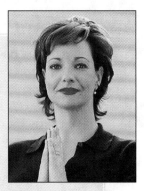

HEALING SPOTLIGHT
Leila Kenzle

Celebrities are people, too. Leila Kenzle, who played Fran Debanow, the wacky best friend on TV's *Mad about You,* has learned her own hard lessons about what works in weight loss—and what doesn't. Here, she talks about the fallacy of gaining comfort from so-called comfort foods.

"I've realized that if I eat the bag of cookies, I'm definitely going to feel worse than I would just dealing with whatever is bothering me. I'm not saying I don't eat chocolate or cookies, but I don't eat them if I'm not okay."

Control Portions

13. Go back to school. Joining a weight-loss class or working with a dietitian can help you learn proper portions, even without weighing and measuring. "If you get ½ cup of cottage cheese, it should look like a tennis ball; ¼ cup should look like a Ping-Pong ball," says Kathy. "Now, I know what appropriate portions look like."

14. Don't toss those measuring cups, though. "I usually misjudge portions of salad dressing, mayonnaise, and ice cream," says Therese. "They're really high in fat and calories and cause the most damage if overdone. So I still measure them."

15. Cook for your family, not an army. Victoria, 39, who shed 60 pounds and has kept it off for 5 years, stopped overfeeding her family of four, even with low-fat foods like grilled chicken. "I stopped making six or seven breasts, thinking that everybody had to have two or three," she says. "Now I make just one for each person."

Cook Smart

16. Plan ahead. An empty fridge after a stressful day begs for pizza. The weight-loss winners don't leave meals to chance. Many of them plan their menus a week or more in advance. Others even cook ahead, freezing meals for the week in individual containers.

17. A little dab will do it. If you just can't pass on some high-fat favorites, stick to the most flavorful ones. "A single slice of bacon is enough to flavor eggs or a potato," says Helen, 61, who lost about 51 pounds. Her husband lost more than 150 pounds.

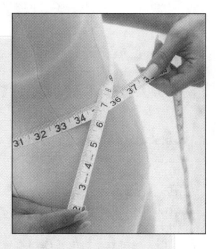

Yes, You Can

Too many of us have little recordings that play in our heads that say something like, "I've never been able to lose weight before, and I won't be able to now. I'm a failure."

That's pretty much writing yourself a script for failure. One way to overcome such negative thinking is to simply turn the tape off. "Pay attention when those self-defeating thoughts pop up," says Joni E. Johnston, Psy.D., a clinical psychologist in Del Mar, California, and author of *Appearance Obsession*. "Every time your internal voice starts saying, 'I'm too fat,' 'I'm too uncoordinated,' 'I can't do it,' answer back, 'That's enough. I can do whatever I put my mind to.'"

18. Fake fry. Try "frying" with calorie-free cooking sprays instead of oil. Spray sliced potatoes and roast them in the oven for french fries that taste fried without the fat, suggests Barbara.

19. Stock frozen veggies. With pasta or stir-fry sauces, they are diet saviors. "I've been known to eat a whole bag of vegetables; and with only ¼ cup of sauce, it's only about 3 grams of fat," says Veronica. "It has saved my butt many times when I was really hungry and had to eat right away."

20. Flavor up. Rice, beans, and other cooked grains are the staples of many successful dieters. For variety, Helen cooks them in different liquids—tomato juice, apple juice, beef or chicken stock. "Rice done in pineapple juice is especially good for rice puddings and Chinese dishes," she says.

Eat Out, but Wisely

21. Be picky. "I'm not afraid to ask for dishes to be prepared differently," says Victoria. "My philosophy is that every restaurant has a grill and an oven. They don't have to fry everything."

22. You'll eat again. This is not your last chance in life to have a particular food. "Those french fries will be there in a ½ hour if I really have to have them," says Veronica. Or they'll be there next week.

23. Don't wait to doggie bag. "As soon as the waitress puts the food down in front of me, I cut the whole portion in half, put it on my

NATURALFACT

The average American swallows at least 20 teaspoons of added sugar (sugar that isn't a natural part of foods) a day.

butter plate, and ask her to wrap it," says Therese. If you wait until the end of your meal, often you pick at it until the waitress returns.

24. Tackle buffets. "I get only 1 tablespoon of everything," says Rebecca. "Usually, I don't even fill my plate, but I at least taste everything so I don't feel deprived."

Trick Temptation

25. Stay busy. Do something that's not conducive to eating. The folks we talked to aren't sitting around thinking of hot-fudge sundaes. They're singing in choirs, taking classes, running marathons, leading weight-loss groups, and more.

26. Keep 'em out of sight. Overwhelmingly, weight-loss vets control foods like chocolate, ice cream, and potato chips by not having them around. "It's easier to fill the house with treats for my kids that I don't like, such as Oreo cookies," says 30-year-old Tammy, who trimmed off 60 pounds.

27. Moderation is key. "If I want a piece of cake, I have one," says Debra, 44, who's 135 pounds slimmer than she was 13 years ago. "Then I just won't have another one for a week or so. Knowing that I can eat something and no one's going to say, 'You can't' works for me."

28. Indulge yourself. Go for the best brand of ice cream or the best cut of steak. "If I'm going to blow 500 or 600 calories, I want to make sure that I'm enjoying it to the max," says Veronica. "Often, desserts look much better than they taste. If it tastes like cardboard, forget it. It's not worth it."

29. Hold back. "When I have to snack, I put my hand in the bag or box and whatever I can grab, that's what I eat—a handful," says Helen.

30. Buy individually packaged snacks. Cookies, chips, even ice cream come in single-serving sizes. "If I want some cookies or chips, I grab one little bag instead of a whole box," says Reed.

31. Remind yourself. A note on the refrigerator reading "Stop" kept Reed from raiding it. Underneath, she listed other things to do, like "Take a drink of water" and questions such as "Are you really hungry?"

32. Find alternatives. Chocolate is still a favorite even for successful dieters. But they've found ways to enjoy it and still keep their waistlines.

Bennett makes fat-free chocolate pudding with skim milk. For Sarah, who lost 40 pounds and has kept it off for 2 years, a cup of sugar-free hot cocoa (about 20 calories), topped with a little fat-free whipped cream does the trick.

33. Don't give in to pressure. If the cookies, chips, or ice cream that you buy for the rest of the family are sabotaging your efforts, stop buying them. "My daughters carried on for about a month, but after that they got used to the change," says Victoria.

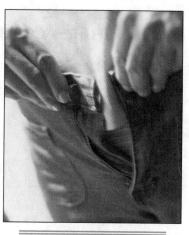

"Even moderate weight losses are beneficial. People don't have to have what seems to be an unattainable goal of losing 50 pounds. If you can lose 15 and keep it off, that's important."

—John Erdman, Ph.D., division of nutritional sciences at the University of Illinois at Urbana-Champaign

Avoid Emotion Eating

34. Know your triggers. You have to know which moods send you to the cookie jar before you can do anything about it. Once you know your triggers, have a list of alternate things to do when the mood strikes. "When I get tired or discouraged, I get an 'I don't care attitude,'" says Rebecca. For those times, taking a walk or reading affirmations can help.

35. Quiz yourself. Determine if you're really hungry or if you're eating for other reasons. "I ask myself, 'Do I really want this, or is it something else, like boredom or depression?' About 80 percent of the time, it's not hunger," says Anne.

36. Call a friend. Talking about what's eating you can keep you from eating. "I had to be willing to call my support people at 9 o'clock on a Friday night," says Barbara, 46, who's kept off 40-plus pounds for more than 15 years.

37. Stop worrying. Remind yourself that you only have control over yourself—not over your spouse, boss, parents, or friends. If you can't do anything about it, just let it go, several people suggested.

38. Take an emotional inventory. Ask yourself, "What do I feel guilty about? Resent? Fear? Regret? What am I angry about?" Then deal with it, says Barbara. Confront the person involved, talk to others, or write a letter—even if you don't send it.

39. Get spiritual. If religion isn't for you, try yoga, meditation, or relaxation exercises. These are especially helpful if you tend to eat when you're stressed, says Barbara.

40. Challenge food. Ice cream is a poor companion if you're lonely. "If I eat the whole bag of chocolate chip cookies, am I going to be any happier? Probably not," says Kathy.

Be Realistic

41. Stay flexible. Many people who have kept the weight off never reached their initial goal weights. Instead, they've gotten to a realistic weight that they can maintain. "In 13 years, I've never gotten down to my initial goal weight, but I'm very happy and feel very good even though I didn't reach it," says Reed.

42. Quit the numbers game. Veronica is 5 feet 5½ inches tall and weighs 152 pounds. By society's standards, she's heavy. However, she can slip into a size 8 thanks to the fact that most of her weight is muscle. "It doesn't matter what the scale says; it matters how I look," she says.

43. Reject others' standards. "Thin is whatever you think thin is. Next to Roseanne Barr, I'm thin. Next to Twiggy, I'm fat," says Barbara.

Take Your Time

To reduce the fat in your diet, it pays to be patient. Studies show that it takes about 3 months to derail any habit—and for most of us, eating fatty foods is a habit.

Get Past Setbacks

44. Stop being a perfectionist. "Look at it like walking a tightrope," suggests Therese. "The goal is not just to stay on without falling off. The goal is to get to the other side, and if you know that you can fall off as many times as you want as long as you get back up again, you're going to be successful."

45. Start fresh. If you have a slip, don't wait until Monday or even tomorrow to get back in line. Therese uses water as a cleansing ritual to end a binge. When she realizes what's happening, she drinks water to signal that the eating is over, and she's back on track immediately. "It's made my lapses shorter and shorter," she says.

46. Practice early detection. "I weigh myself about once a month," says Reed. "If I start inching up, I increase my exercise a little bit."

47. Enlist professional help. Many of the people we talked to used dietitians, personal trainers, and even psychologists to help them deal with problems that were hindering their efforts. If you feel like you can't do it on your own, seek help.

NATURAL HEALING THROUGH HISTORY

In Search of the Perfect Figure

Invent a successful diet today and you're rich, but it wasn't always so.

The robust nudes featured in the seventeenth-century paintings of Peter Paul Rubens, for example, suggest a sensuous appreciation of feminine flesh diametrically opposed to contemporary standards. Calista Flockhart wouldn't qualify.

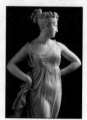

In fact, the shape of the ideal woman has fluctuated dramatically throughout history, according to historian Roberta Pollack Seid, author of *Never Too Thin: Why Women Are at War with Their Bodies*. The ancient Greeks, for example, worshiped a standard of beauty somewhere between that of Rubens' time and our own, as demonstrated by the trim but still roundish contours of their statues. By contrast, paintings around the thirteenth and fourteenth centuries featured women who were thin to the point of starvation. Their appearance was intended to reflect a life of pious self-denial, an image that has been described as holy anorexic. A similar emaciated look became popular again during the Romantic era, when the image of the tortured, starving artist was popularized by such poets as Shelley, Byron, and Keats.

Modern attitudes toward thinness began to evolve during the Enlightenment, Seid says. Reason and refinement came to define the civilized person, which meant that bodily appetites needed to be controlled. Tiny female waistlines became fashionable and have remained that way up until the present day. Breasts and butts, though, were a different story. For most of the nineteenth century, women struggled mightily to achieve the odd proportions of the "hourglass" figure, as the famous corset-cinching scene in *Gone with the Wind* suggests. Other women of Scarlett O'Hara's era sought a more permanent solution. They had their ribs broken or even removed to conform.

Obsessive? Probably, but Seid points out that such concerns were limited mainly to prosperous city girls looking for husbands. In rural women, a heartier build was a sign of robust good health. A male suitor in the 1850s, for example, took out a personal ad seeking a "medium-size, well-developed, erect, and plump" companion. To make sure there were no misunderstandings, he added, "I do not admire skeletons."

Slimness came back into vogue early in the twentieth century, Seid says, courtesy of modern technology. You don't need bulk to run a dishwasher or to drive a car. The modern woman is built to be as strong, efficient, and sleek as the machinery she uses.

Chapter 17

The Secrets to Staying with It

Motivation is the name of the game— here's how to stay on the weight-loss path

Despite the claims of diet hucksters, losing weight is not an overnight proposition. Staying on a weight-loss program is vital—and not always easy. We start out with all the enthusiasm and commitment in the world, but all too soon, we're making excuses or complaining. Before we know it, we're right back where we started.

It doesn't have to be this way. The path to victory isn't as steep as it sometimes seems, and it *is* possible to climb it with careful planning and some advice from the motivation pros.

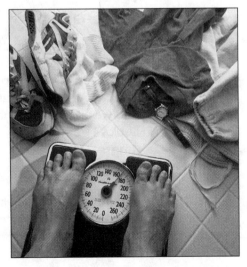

You may notice that some of the experts' tips here were incorporated—intuitively and in some pretty creative ways—by the everyday folks featured in the previous chapter. That might mean that these ideas actually work.

Taking Manageable Steps

Like setting out for a distant destination without a map, setting a goal does not in itself offer clues about how to get where you're going. For more motivation, set a series of short-term goals that break your weight-loss task into achievable sections, giving you a strategy that leads to your long-term objective.

Here's how to set goals and some strategies for making them work.

Be reasonable. Saying "I'll never eat sugar again" usually lands you in the pantry a week later with a handful of cookies and a big load of guilt, says Susan K. Rhodes, Ph.D., director of research for the weight-management center at the Medical University of South Carolina College of Medicine in Charleston. Try setting a more realistic goal: For the next few weeks, put a reasonable number of cookies into your food plan.

Make goals specific. Effective goals define not only what you plan to do but also how, where, and when you'll do it, such as, "At least four times this week, I'm going to try to write down my meals before I eat them."

Focus goals on behavior. Beware of the "I'm going to lose a pound this week" trap. You can't guarantee yourself a weight change. What you can say is, "I'm going to walk every day this week" or "I'm going to nibble on carrots rather than chocolate this week."

Aim goals high. A weight-loss goal that's too difficult will make you want to give up. A goal that's too easy may not get you anywhere. At first, set modest goals that you can achieve quickly, such as switching from whole milk to

Dodge the Bullet

Feeling assaulted by cravings for fatty foods? Here are two ways to avoid the danger, from Linda Crawford, eating-behavior specialist at Green Mountain at Fox Run, a health and weight-management community for women in Ludlow, Vermont.

1. Procrastinate. When you feel compelled to have a fatty food, wait 10 minutes. If you are not really hungry, the craving will pass, Crawford says.

2. Create a diversion. When you feel a craving coming on, distract yourself by engaging in an activity that requires concentration and prevents eating. Take a walk, ride your bike, polish your nails, or play with the kids, says Crawford.

The Weight of History

The average woman carries about 8 percent more body fat than the average man. Why? It's a long story. Prehistoric, in fact.

In caveman days (we'd say "caveperson days," but this was *way* before women's lib), breeding was the primary female career. Often, the males would be off hunting for days at a time, leaving the women with little else but body fat for nourishment. Natural selection favored the survival—and evolution—of females with extra fat cells. Those fat cells protected not only the women but also the unborn children. And, therefore, the species.

1% milk. Then begin to set more ambitious goals, such as switching to fat-free milk.

Write down your goals. Seeing your goals on paper, where you can update them, will make them seem more real and boost your motivation to achieve them, says Virginia Bass, a time-management consultant and owner of By Design, a personal and professional development company in Exton, Pennsylvania, who teaches executives to do this for all kinds of goals. So put your mini-goals on paper, then give yourself a star once you accomplish them. Or make a formal contract with a buddy. Include your goal and the reward for reaching it.

Mentally visualize goals. Close your eyes and picture yourself accomplishing your week's goals. If your mini-goal is to get up 15 minutes earlier to walk the dog, for instance, in your mind, see the alarm clock set at 6:15 A.M. instead of 6:30. See Spot at your bedside with his tail wagging. See your sweats and walking shoes next to the bed, where you placed them the night before. Picture yourself getting into them and getting out there. Now you're set to really do it.

Give yourself a reward. It's important to recognize your achievement when you've reached a goal, and there's no better way to do that than with a reward. Ideally, rewards should be simple, short-term things that you would like to have or do and that don't take a lot of time or money. Try taking a mineral bath, gathering a bouquet of fresh flowers, calling a friend for a long chat, or reading a chapter of a novel that you never seem to have time to finish.

Maintaining Momentum

You can capitalize on the motivation you feel at the beginning of a weight-loss adventure by making some careful plans for later in your fat-fighting journey. Here are some details to remember.

Do a cost-benefit analysis. Divide a sheet of paper into two vertical columns. In the left-hand column, list all the benefits of sticking to your weight-loss plan. Some examples: "I've already dropped 6 pounds," "I have more energy," "I deal with stress better." Under those items, jot down the costs of not sticking to the program, like "I'll be out of shape" or "My belly will come back."

Then, in the right-hand column, write the costs of following your program, such as "I have to cut back on favorite foods that are loaded with fat" or "I have to make time for exercise." Then include the benefits of abandoning the program, such as, "I'll have more time to myself because I won't be walking every day" or "I'll be able to eat and drink whatever I want."

The things in the left column are the thoughts that will motivate you, says Joyce D. Nash, Ph.D., clinical psychologist in San Francisco and Palo Alto, California, and author of *The New Maximize Your Body Potential.* "When your thoughts start drifting to the right column, to the costs of making the changes and the benefits of not bothering, that undermines your motivation."

Post the list where you can see it, as both a visual and mental reminder, every day. Being honest and open about your negative thoughts can help you figure out why you're starting to feel burned out, says Dr. Nash.

Check your records. At the beginning of your fat-fighting journey, write down your weight, body measurements, cholesterol levels, blood pressure, and any other vital statistics. Also write down the amount of time you spend exercising. Then later, if your motivation wanes, check out your progress. Avoid thinking about how far you have to go to reach your

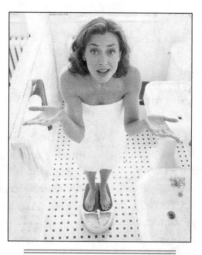

Trying to lose weight because others want you to creates a commitment that may cause feelings of resentment.

long-term weight-loss goals. Instead, pat yourself on the back for the progress that you have made.

Start for the right reasons. Perhaps you decide to lose weight because someone wants you to. Maybe your husband wants you to slim down, or the family doctor keeps pushing the issue, or your mom has been nagging you. Well, ignore them.

"Trying to lose weight because others want you to creates a commitment that may cause feelings of resentment," says Susan J. Bartlett, Ph.D., associate director of clinical psychology at the Johns Hopkins Weight Management Center in Baltimore, and resentment can weaken your resolve. Telling yourself that you "have to" or "should" lose weight, exercise, or stay away from particular foods brings up a rebellious twin who says, "I don't want to have to."

Write down all of the reasons that you decided to eat lower-fat foods and exercise. Each sentence must start with the words "Because I choose to. . . ." When things occasionally get tough, refer to the list.

List your high-risk situations and your defense strategy. Maybe you tend to overeat at restaurants or you have an aversion to working out in cold weather or you have trouble stopping at just two nonfat oatmeal-raisin cookies. Write each of your most tempting situations on the front of a three-by-five index card. Then think of as many counterstrikes as you can and note them on the backs of the cards.

For example, drink a glass of water and have a carrot or celery stalk to take the edge off your hunger before you leave for the restaurant. Try mall walking or gym workouts in the winter. Buy individually wrapped snacks, such as nonfat granola and fruit bars, to keep you from going on a binge. With your defense at the ready, you'll be equipped to handle anything and stay motivated right to the weight-loss finish line.

When the Going Gets Tough

Once you are well into your fat-fighting plan, you may still experience some motivational peaks and valleys. Often, you can link dips to boredom. Here are ways to liven up your routine.

Go on a food safari. Instead of making yourself as miserable as possible by forcing yourself to eat the blandest low-fat foods you can find, think of eating low-fat as a food adventure. Try different recipes. Try different low-fat foods. One low-fat brand of cheese may not taste as dry as another. One vegetarian chili recipe may taste meatier than another. The key is to try a wide variety of low-fat foods.

NATURALFACT

A survey of 83 men and 273 women who had regained weight found that 83 percent of them had reverted to old eating habits and 82 percent had quit their exercise routines.

Change your workout routine. Take your act on the road. Instead of stationary cycling, traverse wooded trails on a mountain bike. Walk in a new area or with a new partner. Try a workout in the morning instead of waiting until the afternoon. Take up a new sport or switch from weight-lifting machines to a free-weight workout.

Or experiment with interval training: After a 10- to 15-minute warmup, step up your pace for about 2 minutes. Slow down to catch your breath, recovering for about 1 minute, then speed up again for another 2. Vary your workouts as much as you like in order to keep them fresh and exciting.

Break up your exercise session. Some people find exercise less boring if they break it up into numerous short sessions instead of one long, arduous workout. Try walking for 10 minutes before work, 15 minutes at lunch, and 10 minutes after dinner, for instance. Doesn't seem like a 35-minute workout, does it?

Distract yourself. Studies show that fast, upbeat music can help motivate you to exercise and keep you going longer. Other effective tactics include watching television or reading while working out on stationary equipment.

Keeping Weight Off

Once you've lost all the weight you've planned to lose, you take on a new motivational challenge. "During maintenance, there isn't that psychological reward of getting on the scale and seeing a smaller number," points out Judy E. Marshel, R.D., director of Health Resources in Great Neck, New York, and former senior nutritionist for Weight Watchers International. "Now, your goal is to see the same number all the time. For some people, it's not nearly as satisfying."

You can keep your motivation going strong, however, just by switching mental tracks. Now, you no longer have a weight-loss goal, but rather a lifestyle goal. Weight maintenance is a lifetime endeavor.

In order to stay motivated and value your efforts, look for new ways to pat yourself on the back. Each morning as you get dressed, for instance, remind yourself how well your clothes fit. Or each time you get on the scale and the number has not budged, consider the event a cause for celebration.

You may have completed the weight-loss race, but now you are embarking on a new, more challenging adventure. Congratulations!

NATURAL HEALING IN THE FUTURE

The Future of Fat

Susan Yanovski, M.D., is the director of the obesity and eating-disorders program of the National Institutes of Health and a member of the National Task Force on Prevention and Treatment of Obesity. Here, she discusses recent developments in

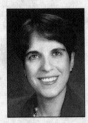 weight-loss research, and where she expects the field to go in the future.

Q: What have been the most important developments in the field of obesity and weight control over the past 5 to 10 years?

A: Certainly, you have to include the better understanding we're developing of some of the genetic and hormonal factors that control how our bodies regulate weight. This can help in understanding why people eat, when they eat, what they eat, why their metabolism is what it is, and what we can do to intervene when it goes awry.

Q: Will this result in more effective treatments?

A: Yes, and hopefully in prevention, too. One of the things that we're learning is that all obesity is not alike. People often think that something is either genetic or behavioral. Behavior can be genetic, too. We don't know as much about that. For example, why do some people eat frequently and get hungry 2 hours after a meal while other people can go 5 hours? Why are some people more physically active than others? If we can learn what's genetic and what's not, then we can look for ways to intervene in those behaviors that are amenable to change.

Q: What other areas are yielding results?

A: We're going from talking about "obesity" to talking about "the obesities." There are a variety of reasons that people become overweight. One exciting area is why some people gain weight more readily than others. The fidgeting study from the Mayo Clinic in Rochester, Minnesota, was an example. It showed that the big difference in weight gain between two normal groups of people was largely dependent on the amount of energy they expended doing things such as maintaining posture, standing, normal walking, and fidgeting. Everyday activities accounted for real differences in energy expenditure.

These are behaviors that people may want to target to prevent weight gain or to keep off lost weight. For example, putting away the remote control and getting up to change the channel every time. Instead of finding ways to conserve energy, such as with the remote, we can find ways to spend energy, such as getting up off the couch and changing the station ourselves. Every little bit helps, particularly for avoiding weight gain.

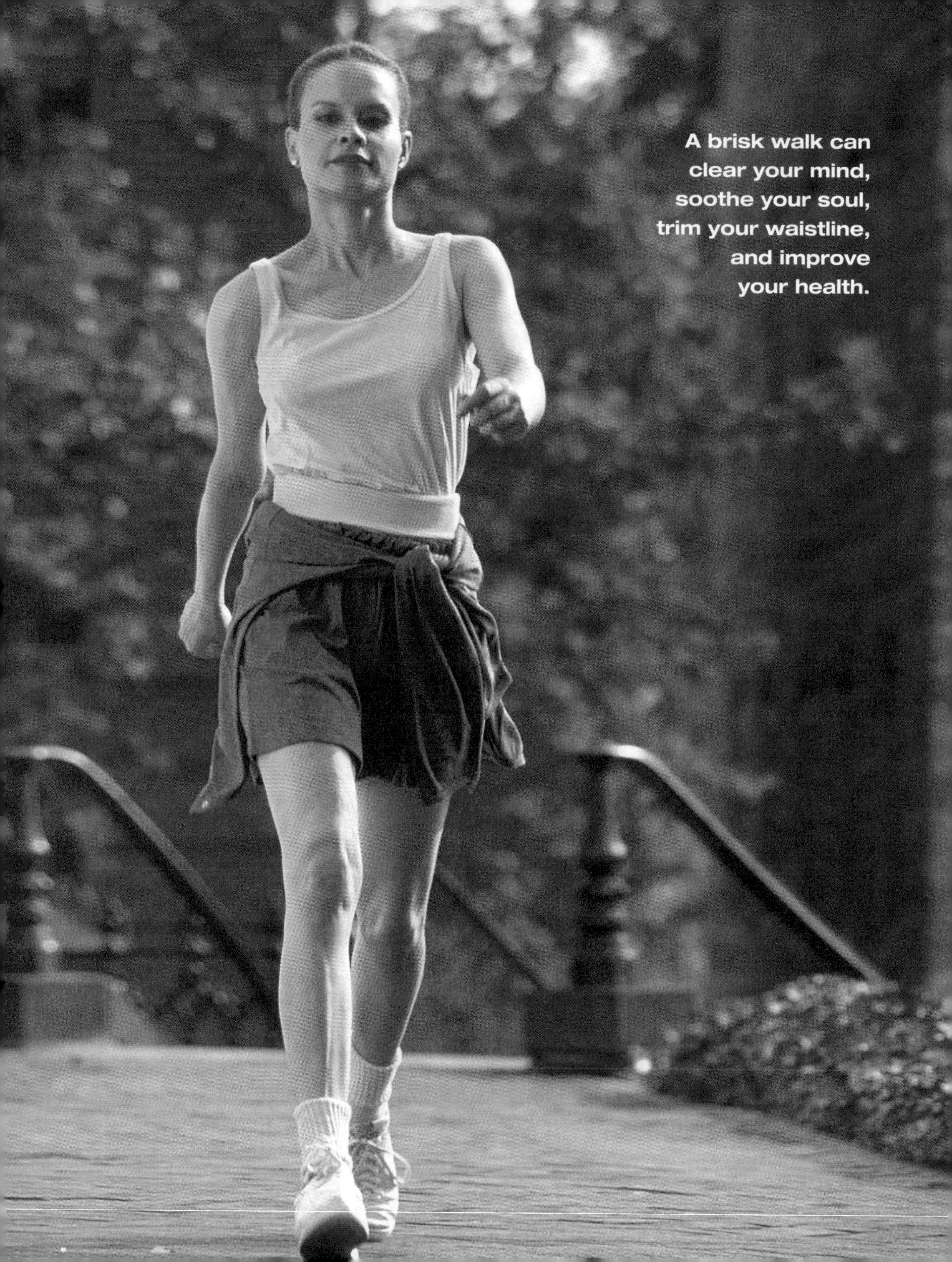

A brisk walk can
clear your mind,
soothe your soul,
trim your waistline,
and improve
your health.

Part Seven

Fit and **Firm**— Naturally

In heaven, it won't be necessary to exercise.
Even in the real world, though, fitness can be easy and fun.

Chapter 18

Walking: The Civilized Exercise

No noisy gyms, no painful injuries—get fit and live to tell about it

Perhaps weight lifting is not for you. Maybe you've had it with those loud and sweaty aerobics classes, too. You might be one of those people who gets tired even thinking about playing tennis or running.

Ready for a kinder, gentler form of exercise?

Try walking. Walking is not only one of the easiest forms of exercise there is, it's also one of the most accommodating.

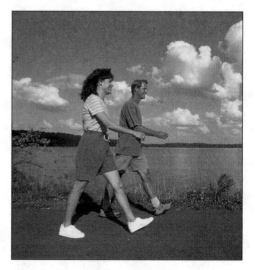

You can think big thoughts while you're walking. Small thoughts, too. You can chat with a friend, walk the dog, or listen to the news on a portable radio. You don't need a gym membership, a trainer, or a scorecard. Just pick a route and be on your way.

Kinder. Gentler. Simpler. What a concept!

How Walking Helps

Given how easy walking is, you might think its health benefits are somewhat limited. You'd be wrong.

Here are a few of the benefits you can enjoy by walking regularly.

- You can lose weight and keep it off.
- Walking can help control diabetes.
- Walking makes your heart stronger, lowers your blood pressure, and boosts levels of good cholesterol in your bloodstream—all of which makes you less susceptible to heart attack and stroke.
- Walking lowers your risk of joint trouble. That's because stronger muscles do a better job of keeping joints in proper alignment, thereby reducing the joint wear and tear that contributes to osteoarthritis.
- Some studies suggest that walking can keep your bones strong, helping you avoid osteoporosis.
- Walking reduces the production of stress hormones, thereby easing depression and anxiety. You feel calmer and happier.

Safe at Any Speed

Unlike other sports, you can build up your level of exercise with walking without ending up in a body cast for 6 months. "The injury rate for walking is far lower than for virtually any other activity," says

Stretching for Walkers

As gentle as it is, walking is still exercise, and as such can put stress on ligaments, tendons, and joints. Here are some warmup stretches that will help keep you walking without pain.

Hip stretch. While standing with your feet shoulder-width apart, step forward with your right foot about 12 inches. Tuck your buttocks under your hips and pull in your stomach muscles. You should feel a stretch at the front of your upper left hip and your upper left thigh. Hold for 15 seconds, then repeat on the other side. You may want to hold on to a table, a tree, or other sturdy object for support.

Shin saver. While standing, cross your left leg over your right. Bend your left knee, pointing your foot like a ballerina so that only the toe of your shoe touches the ground. Then bend your right knee and press your right shin into your left calf.

You should feel a mild stretch in your left shin, says Carol Espel, an exercise physiologist in Westchester, New York. Hold for 15 seconds, then reverse legs and repeat the move. Again, you may want to hold on to something sturdy for balance.

Perfect Walking Posture

Good walking posture helps prevent injuries. To check your technique, have a friend watch you walk, or walk on a treadmill in front of a mirror. Following are the key points of good posture, according to Suki Munsell, Ph.D., founder of the Dynamic Health and Fitness Institute in Corte Madera, California.

Look 6 feet in front of you.

Keep your head level; ears should be over shoulders.

Relax your arms and swing them forward as if they were pendulums.

Drop your shoulders.

Bend your elbows to an 85- to 90-degree angle.

Don't let your hands come across your body.

Keep your abs firm but not so tight that you can't breathe.

Tuck your pelvis slightly by bringing your belly button back toward your spine.

Point your knees and toes forward, keeping your feet parallel.

Roll from heel to toe; avoid falling to the inside or outside of your foot.

Push off with your back foot.

John Duncan, Ph.D., professor of clinical research at Texas Woman's University in Denton and the author of several studies on walking.

That's because walking is a low-impact sport. One of your feet is always on the ground. No bouncing. No pounding. That's good news for your joints and for the vertebrae in your back. For that reason, walking is a particularly good exercise choice if you have arthritis or if you're overweight, since extra pounds also put extra stress on your joints. The same goes for anyone who suffers from lower-back pain. "Walking will strengthen your back muscles without giving your disks a drubbing," says Carol Espel, an exercise physiologist in Westchester, New York.

Trial Run

According to an ancient Chinese adage, "a journey of a thousand miles must begin with a single step." Here are some of the basic rules of walking to help you get started.

Start slowly. Spend the first 5 minutes of each walk just ambling along at your normal walking pace, says Espel. No strain or huffing and puffing. This will give your muscles an opportunity to warm up before you make demands on them. That's important because cold muscles are more vulnerable to exercise-related injuries.

Do some stretches. Once you've loosened up, give your muscles a good stretch to avoid injury. See "Stretching for Walkers" on page 179 for some simple warmup stretches.

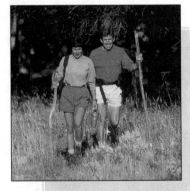

Keep It Interesting

Here are some ways to overcome periods of boredom or stagnation in your walking program.

Take an alternate route. A change of scenery can inspire you. Walk somewhere beautiful such as a hiking trail, along a river, or in a park.

Savor your mileage. As you pick up speed, you'll go farther. Keep a log to track your improvements. Then reward yourself when you top last week's mileage entry.

Sign up for a walking trip. Plan a walking vacation to gorgeous places like the lush, green New England countryside or the sunny California coast. The anticipation will keep you walking.

Be self-indulgent. Walks are your very own time. Relax, take deep breaths, dream, even problem-solve. There are no piles of laundry or ringing phones to distract you.

Pick up the pace. Now you're ready to walk again. Pick up the pace gradually. Don't worry if you're not as fast as the next guy. The important thing when you're starting out is to choose a comfortable pace. You'll pick up speed in due time. "You don't need to huff and puff at first," says Espel. "Walking should be enjoyable, not stressful or painful."

Go around the block. If the last walk you took was down the aisle at your wedding, start short. Walk around the block or, if you're in the country, past four telephone poles. You want to start with a distance that will take you about 10 minutes to cover, notes Espel. Do it three times a week. Remember: Walk at a comfortable pace.

Walk farther. When walking for 10 minutes or so three times a week is no longer a challenge, add distance. Make it 12 to 15 minutes at a pop, Espel says. Gradually work up to 30 minutes three times weekly, then shoot for 30 minutes five times weekly.

If you want to lose weight, shoot for 40 to 60 minutes 4 or 5 days a week, says Dr. Duncan.

Walk faster. Over time, you'll find that you can pick up your pace and still feel comfortable. A good rule of thumb: Walk fast enough that you can talk but not sing. To get all of the cardiovascular benefits that walking offers, Dr. Duncan says, you have to walk at a pace of at least 3 miles an hour, which is about a strolling pace. So make that your minimal goal. If you continue to pick up the pace, the benefits are compounded.

> **NATURALFACT**
>
> Many major thoroughfares built in the United States after World War II aren't walker friendly. Until recently, transportation engineers referred to pedestrians as "traffic flow interruptions."

Get small. The secret to walking faster, oddly enough, is taking smaller steps. "Most people think that to move faster, they should take longer strides, but quicker, shorter steps make you move faster," explains Espel. That's because your hips can rotate faster when you shorten your stride. And if you pump your arms faster, your feet have to follow.

Cool your heels. Cool down by spending the last 5 minutes of your walk strolling, says Espel.

Stretch again. Finally, follow your cooldown with some basic stretches so that you don't become stiff and rigid. Stretching after a workout is, if anything, more important than stretching before. You can repeat the stretches that you did to warm up, plus a few more.

Foot roll. This gives your hardworking shins and calves a good after-walk stretch. Stand with your feet 6 to 12 inches apart, then slowly roll up onto your toes and hold for a count of two. Then roll over onto the outsides of your feet and hold for two. Next, roll back onto your heels and lift your toes. Hold for a count of two. Finish with your feet flat on the ground. Repeat up to 10 times.

Caution: Rolling your feet and ankles can lead to injury if you're not careful—you may want to hold on to something sturdy for balance.

Back relaxer. Lie on your back with your knees bent. Place your left hand on the outside of your left thigh (about midthigh) and your right hand on the outside of your right thigh and pull your knees toward your chest. Hold for 15 seconds.

Hamstring stretch. Lie on your back and bend your left knee so the foot is flat on the floor. Extend your right leg straight up toward the ceiling, keeping your back and hips on the floor. Hold the stretch for 15 to 30 seconds and then switch legs.

Two Walking Workouts

It always helps to have a plan. We have two.

The two walking workout plans below were designed by Rebecca Gorrell, director of fitness and movement therapy at Canyon Ranch in Tucson. Follow them faithfully, and you'll go from being a beginner to an experienced walker. Not incidentally, you'll shed some pounds along the way.

The Get-Started Plan

Even though we all do some walking in the course of our day-to-day lives—to the bathroom, the bedroom, and the kitchen, if nowhere else— walking for weight loss is something to build up to. When Suzanne, a New York City podiatrist, started walking, the extra pounds she carried made even short workouts feel intense. "I walked at about a 20- to 25-minute-per-mile pace and was huffing and puffing," she says. "Now I do less than a 14-minute mile and walk 4 miles a day."

This program is designed to ease you into a regular walking routine. It's perfect for the absolute beginner, especially for someone who is severely overweight or who currently does little or no exercise. By starting out slowly, you'll enjoy walking more, build your confidence, and reduce your risk of injury. Even at a slow pace, you'll reap many benefits. From the start, you'll feel more energetic and flexible, and you'll be in a better mood. After about 2 weeks, your walks

Get-Started Workout

	Duration	Frequency	Intensity	Speed
WEEK 1	10 min.	3 days	Moderate*	Whatever is comfortable
WEEK 2	15 min.	4 days	Moderate*	As if you're in a bit of a hurry; after walking for 10 min., you should have covered more distance than you did last week
WEEK 3	20 min.	5 days	Moderate*	As if you're in a bit of a hurry
WEEK 4	30 min.	5 days	Moderate*	As if you're in a bit of a hurry; enough to get your heart pumping, but not enough to leave you out of breath

*Enough to get your heart pumping, but not enough to leave you out of breath

will feel easier because your heart will be getting fitter and your legs will be getting stronger.

The Keep-Going Plan

This program is designed specifically to keep you walking after the initial charge of starting to get in shape has faded. In particular, it's intended to help you over the infamous workout plateau.

Any regular exerciser is familiar with the plateau phenomenon. That's the point where you seem to be doing the same amount of work but not seeing the same amount of progress. Weight loss may level off; you don't seem to be increasing your distance or speed

The Keep-Going Workout

	Duration	Frequency	Program	Pace
WEEK 1	35 min.	5 days	Warmup (5 min.)	Leisurely stroll
			Normal walk (5 min.)	Steady
			Speedup (5 min.)	Walk as if in a hurry
			Recovery (10 min.)	Steady
			Speedup (5 min.)	Walk as if in a hurry
			Cooldown (5 min.)	Leisurely stroll
WEEK 2	35 min.	5 days	Warmup (5 min.)	Leisurely stroll
			Normal walk (5 min.)	Steady
			Speedup (5 min.)	Walk as if in a hurry
			Recovery (10 min.)	Steady
			Speedup (5 min.)	Walk as if in a hurry
			Cooldown (5 min.)	Leisurely stroll
WEEK 3	45 min.	5 days	Warmup (5 min.)	Leisurely stroll
			Normal walk (5 min.)	Steady
			Speedup (5 min.)	Walk as if in a hurry
			Recovery (8 min.)	Steady
			Speedup (5 min.)	Walk as if in a hurry
			Recovery (7 min.)	Steady
			Speedup (5 min.)	Walk as if in a hurry
			Cooldown (5 min.)	Leisurely stroll
WEEK 4	45 min.	5 days	Warmup (5 min.)	Leisurely stroll
			Speedup (5 min.)	Walk as if in a hurry
			Recovery (5 min.)	Steady
			Speedup (5 min.)	Walk as if in a hurry
			Recovery (5 min.)	Steady
			Speedup (5 min.)	Walk as if in a hurry
			Recovery (5 min.)	Steady
			Speedup (5 min.)	Walk as if in a hurry
			Cooldown (5 min.)	Leisurely stroll

as consistently as you had. It's a frustrating point that causes many exercisers to give up and head back to their TV sets. Don't let this happen to you.

A simple change in your workout can send the plateau blues packing. An excellent way to achieve such a change is to add "intervals" to your workout routine. The idea is to alternate periods of intense effort with short periods of "active rest," in which you keep moving, but at a relatively easy pace. The trick is not to let your heart rate slow all the way down to easy-chair levels during the active rest phase. By pushing yourself to achieve the more intense level of exercise, you'll overcome your plateau—and burn off calories at a blistering pace.

Onward and Upward!

Once you get used to exercising, there's an irresistible temptation to push a little harder each time you go out. Here are some ways to make your walks more challenging.

Hill walking. This is just what it sounds like: walking up and down hills. Repeatedly. Hill walking gives your heart a more strenuous workout. It can also help shape up your tush. To do it, find some moderately steep hills (nothing Himalayan—an incline of about 4 to 8 percent will do) and tread up and down them for 20 minutes.

Interval walking. To do this, you walk as fast as you can for 30 seconds, then, over the next 90 seconds, slow down to your usual pace. Then you go as fast as you can for another 30 seconds and drop down again to your regular pace. And then you do it again. You get the idea.

Interval walking burns more calories and gives your stamina a bigger boost than the regular variety. The Keep-Going Workout is an example of an interval walk.

Distance walking. Walking more than 4 miles at a time qualifies as distance walking, says Carol Espel, an exercise physiologist in Westchester, New York. "This is something you can do when you're preparing for an event, like a 5-K walking race," she explains. Walking races add a competitive element to walking—an extra incentive for Type A personalities. To find out about races in your area (most running races welcome walkers), give a local sporting goods store or YMCA a call.

NATURAL HEALING THROUGH HISTORY

Marilyn Monroe:
Norma Jean's Fitness Routine

Stop for a minute and picture Marilyn Monroe. Is she posing, smiling for the camera, blonde hair rustling in the breeze? Probably. Is she holding a dumbbell? Probably not. Beautiful blondes in the 1950s weren't supposed to sweat.

The secret truth is, though, that Marilyn *did* sweat for the sake of her camera-friendly figure, albeit discreetly. "I'm fighting gravity," she confessed. "If you don't fight gravity, you sag."

So, Marilyn jogged. She began running in the mornings in the 1940s, 30 years before the jogging craze. Possibly in order to avoid fans trying to catch a glimpse of the rising star, in the early 1950s she ran through the alleys of Hollywood before breakfast. Since she was running many years before spandex and sneakers were common, Marilyn ran in jeans and a bralike top.

Behind closed doors where few cameras could spy, Marilyn (born Norma Jean Mortensen) also took up bodybuilding. She began weight lifting in 1943, a few years before her face graced its first magazine cover. She started by taking lessons once a week to learn how to weight lift with small dumbbells. By 1951, she regularly did 40 minutes of calisthenics, plus a workout with two 5-pound dumbbells. One rare photo shows Marilyn lying on her back on a weight bench wearing jeans and a halter

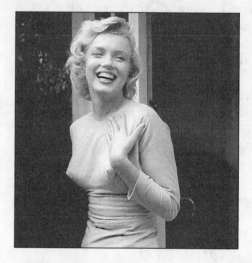

top, coolly bench-pressing two barbells.

In addition to these regimens, Marilyn also enjoyed other fitness activities. She could sometimes be spotted riding her English bicycle in Central Park in New York City or pedaling around Brooklyn's Sheepshead Bay and Coney Island with her third husband, Arthur Miller. Another rare old photo shows her golfing, but it's probably just a pose. She's happily standing in white heels on the putting green.

It's easy to understand why Marilyn felt that she needed to stay in shape. Few women before her had been so prominently on public display, after all, and so revealingly. As a sex goddess, low-cut gowns were part of her working clothes.

Chapter 19

Get In Shape— And Stay That Way

Our no-nonsense program produces results within a week, guaranteed

There are two major problems with getting into shape: It's too hard, and it takes too long.

But what if someone designed an easy-to-follow fitness program that was guaranteed to burn fat and build muscle—a program that would show results in one week? A program that took less than an hour a day?

Sound too good to be true? It's not. We asked one of the top fitness experts in the country—Wayne Westcott, Ph.D., strength consultant to the YMCA of the USA—to design the perfect workout program for us, and he did. This isn't one of those phony "miracle" deals. It's a solid, commonsense exercise program. The great thing is that it works quickly, and anybody can do it.

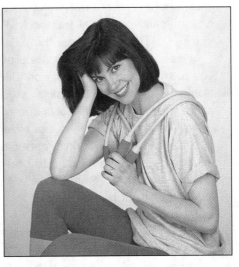

Road-Tested for Success

We know this program works because we road-tested it on 10 real-life women (no ringers from the world of professional bodybuilders). How'd they do?

Even better than we'd hoped. Each week, they lost an average of 1½ pounds and gained about ¾ pound of muscle. That's a 9-pound change in body composition in just 4 weeks.

Some did even better. One of our test subjects, a woman in her midforties, lost 9 pounds of fat while building 5 pounds of muscle, for a grand total body composition change of 14 pounds.

That's pretty good—and far from impossible. You can achieve the same results—and you'll see noticeable progress within a week.

One warning: Don't be discouraged if you work out for a few weeks and discover that you've actually *gained* weight. Muscle weighs more than fat. In fact, a handful of muscle tissue is 22 percent heavier than the same size handful of fat. So as you increase muscle and decrease fat, you won't see a drastic change on the scale. What counts is that muscle takes up less space. It also looks a heck of a lot better. For a more accurate measure of your progress, have your body fat percentage measured (you can do this at most health clubs). Or take tape measurements of your waist, hips, and thighs. Chances are you'll be very pleasantly surprised with what you see.

Now, let's get started!

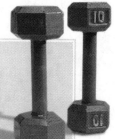

What to Expect

Follow our workout program, and you'll be amazed at how quickly your body responds. Week by week, you can expect these results.

Week 1: You'll increase the amount of weight you're lifting and feel more confident. "I was having trouble balancing while doing lunges at first. Now I'm much more in control," says one of our test subjects, Lisa Getz. "It feels like my legs have come out of hibernation and are alive again."

Week 2: You'll get firm, especially in your arms and calves, and feel stronger. "It's so rewarding to see myself get stronger so quickly," says test subject Naomi Betancourt, who wants to get back into a size 8. "I love the definition in my arms."

Week 3: You'll lose pounds and inches. Lisa, who wanted to get in shape for her upcoming wedding, lost nearly 4 pounds and 2½ inches in just 3 weeks.

Week 4: You'll see a slimmer, firmer body. "I'm feeling good and my energy level is up!" says Naomi.

Work Out Wisely

Here are a few basics you should know before starting a strength-training program.

- **Pick the right weight.** Choose a weight you can lift 10 to 15 times while maintaining good form. If you can easily do more than 15 repetitions ("reps," in gymspeak), the weight is too light.
- **Power up for faster results.** When you can easily do 15 reps, increase the amount of weight you're lifting in 10 percent increments.
- **Breathe properly.** Inhale as you lower weights with gravity and exhale as you lift against it.
- **Go slowly.** You'll get much more value out of lifting if you don't rush it. Each repetition should take about 6 seconds. Slowly count 1-2-3 as you lift the weight and 1-2-3 as you lower it.
- **Protect your back.** Don't put yourself at risk for back pain. Always squat and lift with your legs when picking up weights, rather than bending forward and lifting with your back.

The Program

You will need two sets of dumbbells (5 pounds and 10 pounds), one set of adjustable ankle weights (up to 10 pounds a leg), and a bench. That's all.

The program consists of just three elements.

- An upper-body workout, done twice a week
- A lower-body workout, also done twice a week
- An aerobic activity, done six days a week

The aerobic activity lasts half an hour and includes a wide variety of options, from walking and swimming to cycling or an aerobics class. The 30 minutes includes warmup, cooldown, and stretching—all necessary to avoid injury. Here's how a sample week might go.

Monday: Aerobics, upper-body workout
Tuesday: Aerobics, lower-body workout
Wednesday: Aerobics
Thursday: Aerobics, upper-body workout
Friday: Aerobics, lower-body workout
Saturday: Aerobics
Sunday: Rest

Here are the workouts.

Upper-Body Workout

Each upper-body workout consists of 10 to 15 repetitions—one "set"—of each of the following nine exercises.

You'll do two of these workouts a week. Muscles need a day's rest in between workouts, which is why you should do upper-body and lower-body workouts on alternate rather than consecutive days.

After 2 weeks, increase to two sets of each exercise.

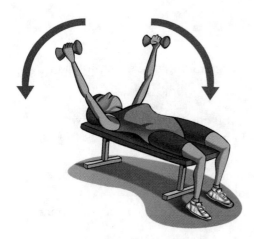

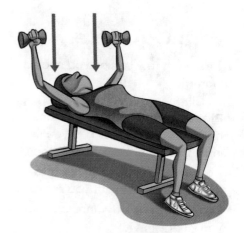

1. Chest fly: Lie on your back on a bench. Hold the dumbbells above your chest with your palms facing each other and elbows slightly flexed. Lower your arms downward and out to the sides, keeping your elbows slightly flexed. Stop when your upper arms are parallel to the floor. Return to the starting position.

2. Chest press: Hold the dumbbells over your chest so the ends face each other and your palms are facing the ceiling. Lower your arms so that your elbows point toward the floor and the weights are even with your chest. Return to the starting position.

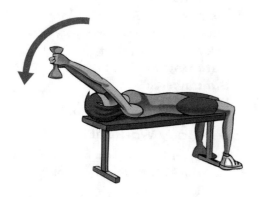

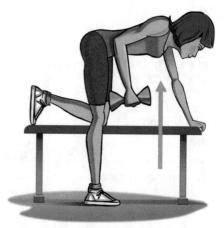

3. Dumbbell pullover: Hold one dumbbell with both hands above your upper chest. Lower your arms downward and backward over your head as far as possible without discomfort. Return to the starting position. Don't arch your back.

4. Bent-over row: With your left knee on the bench and your right foot on the floor, hold a dumbbell with your right hand. Let your arm hang straight down with your palm facing the bench. Pull the dumbbell up to your chest, and then lower. Repeat on the other side.

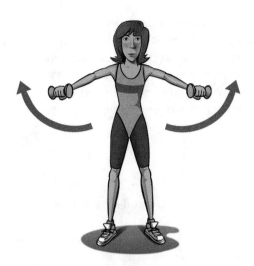

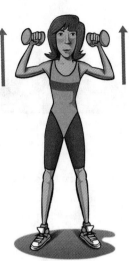

6. Shoulder press: Start with the dumbbells at shoulder height, palms facing in. Press the dumbbells straight up overhead and then lower. Don't arch your back.

5. Lateral raise: Hold the dumbbells at your sides, with your elbows slightly bent. Raise the dumbbells outward until your arms are parallel to the floor, then lower.

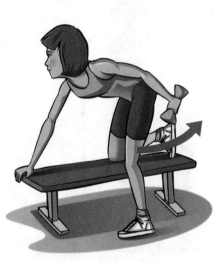

7. Biceps curl: Hold the dumbbells at your sides. Keeping your elbows at your sides, lift the dumbbells upward. Turn your wrists so the dumbbells end up at chest height, palms facing your chest, then lower.

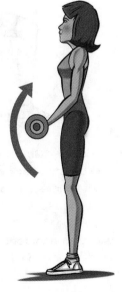

8. Triceps kickback: With your right knee on the bench and your left foot on the floor, grasp a dumbbell with your left hand. Start with your elbow at your side so your forearm is perpendicular to the floor. Move your hand backward, bending your arm at the elbow, until your forearm is parallel to the floor. Lower to the starting position. Repeat with your right arm.

(continued)

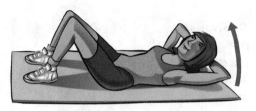

9. Abdominal crunch: Lie on a carpeted floor with your knees bent and your feet flat on the floor. Place your hands loosely behind your head. Slowly curl your shoulders about 3 inches off the floor, then slowly lower to the floor.

Lower-Body Workout

The routine is the same: Do 10 to 15 repetitions (one set) of each of these nine exercises twice a week.

Again, don't do this workout on consecutive days; your muscles need a day's rest in between.

And again, increase your workout to two sets of each exercise after 2 weeks.

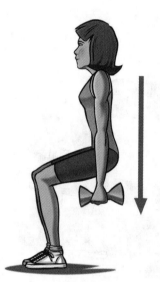

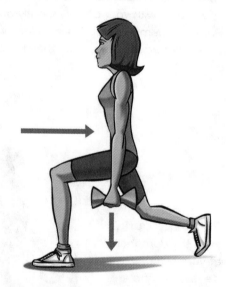

1. Squat: Stand against a wall, holding a dumbbell in each hand. Keep your head up, shoulders back, and back straight; slide down as if sitting in a chair. Don't go lower than having your thighs parallel to the floor; don't let your knees move forward over your toes. Return to the starting position.

2. Lunge: Grasping the dumbbells, take one big step back with your right leg. Plant your feet, and then slowly lower your right knee toward the floor. Your left knee should be at a 90-degree angle. Push off with your right foot, and return to the starting position. Repeat with your left leg.

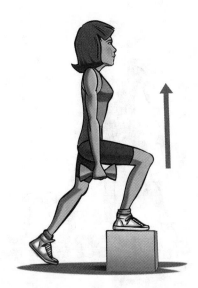

4. Hip flexion: With ankle weights on, stand behind a chair, lightly holding on to it for support. Bring your right knee up until your thigh is parallel to the floor. Return to the starting position. Repeat with your left leg.

3. Step up: Hold your dumbbells at your sides. Step up with your right leg, followed by your left leg, so both feet are on the step. Then step down with your right foot, followed by your left. Repeat, starting with your left leg.

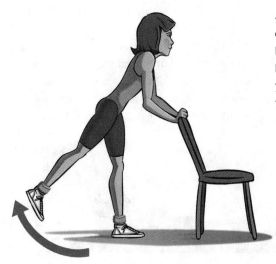

5. Hip extension: With ankle weights on, stand about 18 inches behind a chair. Bend 45 degrees at your waist, lightly holding on to the chair for support. Lift your right leg straight behind you until your leg and torso are in a straight line, and then lower. Repeat with your left leg.

(continued)

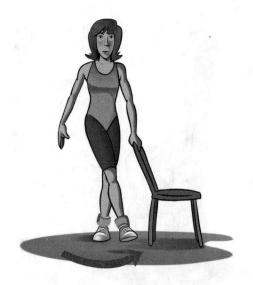

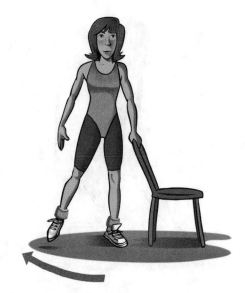

6. Hip adduction: With ankle weights on, stand to one side of a chair, lightly holding on for support. Lift your right leg across the front of your body at about a 45-degree angle. Lower. Repeat with your left leg.

7. Hip abduction: Start in the same position as for the hip adduction. Then lift your right leg out to the side and lower. Repeat with your left leg.

8. Calf raise: With dumbbells in hand, stand with your legs about hip-width apart. Slowly rise up onto your toes while keeping your torso erect and your knees straight. Hold, then lower.

9. Trunk extension: Lie facedown on a carpeted floor with your forehead on the floor and your hands behind your head. Using your lower-back muscles, slowly lift your head and chest off the floor. Hold, and then lower. To make this exercise easier, place your palms flat on the floor near your head for assistance when rising.

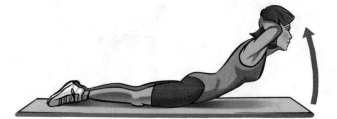

NATURAL HEALING IN THE FUTURE

The New Benefits of Exercise

Miriam Nelson, Ph.D., is associate chief of the physiology laboratory at Tufts University in Boston and author of the best-selling book *Strong Women Stay Young*. She also writes a monthly column on strength training for *Prevention*.

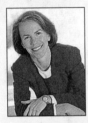

Q: What have been the most exciting developments in fitness and exercise over the past 5 to 10 years?

A: Three areas are particularly interesting. The first is the research on physical activity improving longevity and reducing disease risk. We now have a number of very large studies showing that physical activity—any physical activity—increases longevity and decreases risk of heart disease, diabetes, and osteoporosis. And this is true even if you smoke or are overweight.

The next one is the importance of strength training such as weight lifting, which builds muscle. As we grow older, we lose muscle and become weaker, making even everyday tasks more difficult. As a result, strength training becomes more and more important, for women in particular. We're not as strong as men; we don't have as much muscle or bone. That's why it's even more important for us to optimize and preserve what we have.

The third area is the mind/body connection with physical activity. For years we focused on body fat, muscle strength, and cardiovascular health. Now research is showing how important physical activity is to improving self-confidence, self-esteem, and body image; reducing depression, anxiety, and stress; and improving sleep.

Q: What breakthroughs or changes can we expect to see in the next 5 to 10 years?

A: I saw a news report recently about an adult exercise class called Recess. It's total fun play. We have to come up with more types of fun exercise. The more variety there is, the more options people will have.

The trouble is that we have a work culture that doesn't embrace physical activity. Even for me, it's hard. We brought in a tai chi instructor. Once a week at 1:00 P.M. on Thursdays, we all feel guilty because we're at our tai chi class—and we're an exercise physiology lab! This work culture is going to kill us.

Another important area we'll be addressing in the future is specificity. Even the healthiest people, regardless of what age they are, have certain things that they need to work on more than others. The tall, slender woman is very different from the short, stocky woman. If your father died early of heart disease and your mother has diabetes, your exercise prescription would be very different from mine if my mother had osteoporosis and breast cancer.

Depending on your goals, your family history, and your time commitments, you'll be able to figure out the best exercise program for you.

**Letting little
things upset you
can mean a
greater risk
of heart disease.**

Part Eight

Your
Emotions
and Your
Health

*The mind-body revolution shows that health
and happiness are intimately connected.*

Chapter 20

Plug Into the Mind-Body Connection

You are what you eat—*and* what you think, what you feel, and what you believe

If you doubt that your thoughts and emotions have an impact on what happens in your body, try this. Put your hand flat on a table. Lift your index finger.

Now, picture in your mind a sexual fantasy. Pay attention to your body's changes.

Both of these activities demonstrate that the mind and body do indeed interact with one another, constantly and intimately. That's the essence of the mind-body connection.

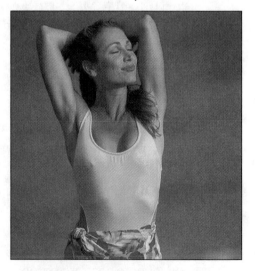

Research has shown that this mind-body duet has a far greater impact on our health and our emotions than we ever imagined, and those discoveries are changing the face of medicine as we've known it.

Here's a look at what the mind-body revolution is all about.

Emotional Molecules

Not so long ago, scientists believed that the mind and the immune system operated relatively independently of one another. We now know that that assumption was false. Researchers have discovered that there are nerves that connect the immune system to the nervous system, which, in turn, is directly wired to the brain. They have also discovered neuropeptides, molecules that carry messages between the brain and every cell in the body, enabling them to communicate constantly with one another.

Numerous experiments have verified the effects of this chemical exchange. One study, conducted at Ohio State University in Columbus, showed that students have weaker immune systems during final exams.

Another study, conducted at the University of California, Los Angeles, found that actors could cause changes in their immune systems merely by pretending to experience happiness or sadness when asked to think of various scenarios.

What this means is that emotions can have a direct impact on the body's defenses against disease, theoretically making us more or less susceptible to everything from the common cold to AIDS. "The mental is physical, and the physical is mental," says Candace Pert, Ph.D., research professor of physiology and biophysics at Georgetown University Medical Center in

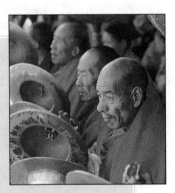

Mind over Matter

It makes sense to be skeptical of snake charmers and mind readers in carnival sideshows. When an associate professor of medicine at Harvard Medical School starts talking about miraculous feats of mind over matter, though, it makes sense to listen.

The professor in question is Herbert Benson, M.D., a pioneer in mind-body medicine and president of the Mind/Body Medical Institute at New England Deaconess Hospital in Boston. In his book *Timeless Healing*, Dr. Benson describes visits that he and his team of researchers made to the Himalayas to study the meditation techniques of Tibet's Buddhist monks.

"Our teams documented that monks could indeed dry icy, wet sheets on their naked bodies in temperatures of 40 degrees Farenheit," Dr. Benson writes. "Within 3 to 5 minutes of applying the dripping 3-by-6-foot sheets to their skin, the sheets began to steam! Within 20 to 40 minutes, the sheets were completely dry, and they were able to repeat this process two more times."

Washington, D.C., and author of the book *Molecules of Emotion: Why You Feel the Way You Feel.* "The mind and the body are really inseparable. They're one."

How Anger Hurts

You don't have to look through a microscope in a laboratory to see the truth of the mind-body connection. Researchers have come to identical conclusions by observing thousands of men and women in the real world.

One of the first such studies to gain widespread attention was the identification in the 1960s of the famous type A personality. Two California cardiologists demonstrated that type A men—those who were hurried, competitive, and hostile—were twice as likely to develop heart disease as men who didn't have those characteristics. Subsequent researchers would refine that hypothesis, singling out hostility as the most unhealthy of the type A character traits.

In one study, some 1,300 men in Boston were given a questionnaire designed to determine their predispositions for anger. Possible responses included statements such as "At times, I feel like picking a fistfight" and "I have been so angry that I felt as if I would explode." Those whose test scores were highest were found to be three times more likely to develop heart disease than those with low scores.

Hostility is harmful because it kicks off the fight-or-flight reflex, pumping loads of hormones into the system. The body releases adrenaline, and blood pressure and heart rate increase.

These are all useful if you're dodging a dinosaur out by the watering hole, but they're a little excessive if you're just getting jostled on a city sidewalk.

The fight-or-flight reflex is also kicked off by stress, which probably edges out hostility as the most pervasive of all the modern ills. "I am convinced that stress is a primary cause or aggravating factor in many conditions that bring patients to doctors," says Andrew Weil, M.D., author of the bestselling books *Spontaneous Healing* and *Eight Weeks to Optimum Health*.

Researchers suspect that stress reduces the supply of oxygen to the heart while simultaneously increasing demand for oxygen. People who react strongly to stress have been shown to be three times more likely to have heart attacks or need heart surgery than those who don't.

The Mind-Body Upside

Although a lot of the mind-body research conducted so far has focused on the harmful potential of negative emotions, there's plenty of evidence showing that our feelings can be our allies, too. One of the groundbreaking mind-body studies conducted at Stanford University found that being in a support group helped cancer patients stay in remission and, therefore, live longer.

The message of this study is clear: There are ways that the mind's self-healing potential can be marshaled to overcome less-than-optimal conditions.

One of the leaders in showing how we can do just that is Herbert Benson, M.D., associate professor of medicine at Harvard Medical School and president of the Mind/Body Medical Institute at New England Deaconess Hospital in Boston. Dr. Benson developed the relaxation response, a simple four-step meditation technique that enables patients to lower their blood pressures, heart rates, rates of breathing, and muscle tension. He calls the calming effect of the relaxation response the opposite effect of the fight-or-flight response and says that it can alter the way the body reacts to stress after the exercise has been completed.

This isn't the only such method to have been developed. Techniques as various as yoga, tai chi, and even knitting can elicit the same response. So can exercise and prayer.

A Winning Attitude

Another key to marshaling the body's self-healing resources is attitude. Research has shown that the way we interpret and react to life's trials can determine how they affect our immune systems. One study conducted at the University of Chicago observed 200 telecommunications executives as their company went through a downsizing. Those who survived the transition with their good health intact tended to see change as an opportunity for growth rather than as a threat. They also had strong networks of social support and a deep sense of commitment to their jobs and families. Executives who possessed these qualities of "psychological hardiness" had less than a 33 percent chance of contracting a severe

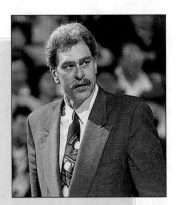

HEALING SPOTLIGHT
Phil Jackson

To be a coach in the National Basketball Association would be enough stress for anyone, but for 10 years, Phil Jackson had the added pressure of leading the fabled Chicago Bulls. Monumental talents, yes. Monumental egos, too. And monumental expectations.

How did Jackson maintain his sanity? Practicing Zen meditation each morning helped.

"Meditation allows you to sit and let the mind realize who's in control," he says. "Thoughts come and go, but you don't let them possess you. It gives you a chance to enter the day with peacefulness and also with compassion. The other reason I meditate is to wake up—to be conscious and alert. One of the things that I teach in basketball is that alertness is the key, so I apply it to that."

illness during or soon after the downsizing process, while executives who didn't possess them had a probability of severe illness that was higher than 9 chances in 10.

Putting Emotions to Use

For all it has to offer, mind-body medicine is not exactly on the road map yet at most standard health clinics or doctor's offices, where the purely physical is still the preferred guide for identifying routes to good health. With some exceptions, mainstream medicine is taking a wait-and-see approach, says Dr. Weil.

But alternative medicine isn't waiting. In fact, the mind-body unity is a given in virtually all alternative modalities, and it is often a central part of their healing philosophy. This isn't to say that you need to see an alternative therapist to put the mind-body connection to work in *your* life.

To the contrary, there are dozens of easy-to-use techniques for improving both your emotional life and your health by simply paying attention to how each of them affects the other.

Chapter 21

"I Defeated My Food Addiction"

"Overeating nearly drove me to suicide, but I fought my inner demons and won"

For some people, it's booze; for others, drugs. For Lynne Watson, it was food.

Eating was the love of Watson's life—until she reached 230 pounds. Her health was falling apart; she felt she was ready to die. She didn't.

Addictions of any kind can drag us down, but this story demonstrates that we *can* break the grip of negative emotions that lead to destructive behaviors. Watson found the courage to change. Controlling her eating was only part of the battle. She also took the difficult steps she had to take in order to clear her life of the things that were crippling her belief in herself. Here's her story.

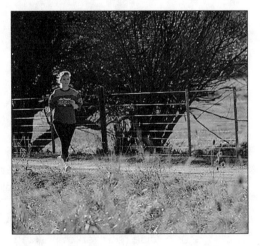

Eating to Ease the Pain

All my life, I'd struggled with my weight; and for the past 3 years, I'd been turning to food for consolation. Eating was my way of dealing with my husband's drinking, and it had become my own sort of addiction. My mornings started at the bakery, where I'd pick up an apple fritter and two or three chocolate doughnuts, which I'd polish off before I got to work. Then, in the evenings, I'd sit down to a Mexican dinner slathered in cheese, sour cream, and guacamole. Eating was basically my only joy.

Some joy. At 230 pounds, I looked and felt terrible. My lower back, joints, and feet ached. I had asthma, poor circulation, chronic constipation, and heartburn. As I sat alone on Christmas Day 1985, I realized that I had two choices: end my life or take control of it. The one thing I couldn't do was go on in the same way. I decided to grab control.

Taking Action

I started by talking to friends, my priest, and even a therapist about getting a divorce. By the spring, I had taken the first tentative steps toward ending my 19-year marriage and returning to school with intentions of completing my bachelor's degree.

As I made these choices, I began to feel empowered. I found I did have a modicum of control over my life—and it was time I exercised it. That's when I decided to lose weight.

I went on a diet. Not a crazy diet—I'd tried every pill, gimmick, and program before—but a sensible, three-meals-a-day diet that cut out between-meal snacks. Breakfast became fruit and cereal, lunch was a frozen Lean Cuisine or Weight Watchers meal, and dinner was a vegetable stir-fry over rice. If I got hungry between meals, I'd have a diet soda and a rice cake.

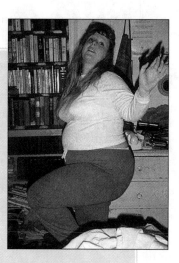

How She Did It

Weight lost: 105 pounds

Time to reach goal: 4 years

Other health benefits: Gained more energy and stamina; improved muscle tone; and relieved asthma symptoms, back, foot, and joint pain, and digestive and circulation problems

Successful strategies: Low-fat, vegetarian diet; an exercise regimen of walking, running, and strength training

Battling Food

I did everything I could to take my mind off food and discovered that it was easier if I got out of the house and away from the fridge. Taking classes helped, and I joined my church choir. As I met new people, I learned to rely on them, rather than food, for comfort and companionship.

I began getting off the bus a mile before my stop each day. From there, I'd trudge up and down the San Francisco hills to my office. In the evening, I'd repeat the process. It wasn't easy. It took me 45 minutes to walk just over a mile, and I had to stop often to catch my breath. But I enjoyed being outdoors. Most of all, I liked the feeling that, finally, I was doing something good for me.

At first, the pounds just disappeared. When my weight loss would slow, I'd shave a few more calories from my diet and add more distance or hills to my route. After a few months, I was walking about 3½ miles a day. Within a year, I was down to 165 pounds. But then I hit a wall.

A Setback Looms

I was having trouble adapting to life as a single person and found myself slipping back into my old ways when the weight loss slowed. When I felt sorry for myself, I'd indulge in pizza or a chocolate chip cookie. I joined a gym, hoping that would get me back on track, but my workouts were halfhearted.

A year went by, and I hadn't lost a pound. I was really discouraged. Then I met Paul. We both loved classical music and hit it off instantly. Knowing that losing weight was important to me, Paul encouraged me to start running in the mornings. I loved this new kind of exercise. It was exhilarating to get up early and run a mile around the track in the park. In the evenings and on weekends, Paul and I would hike in the nearby hills.

Paul is a vegetarian, and I became interested in preparing delicious, healthy, meatless meals. I also discovered that I loved foods like soy burgers. It wasn't long before I gave up meat entirely.

New Husband, New Life

By the time Paul and I were married in 1990, I weighed 119 pounds. (He had also trimmed down from 205 to 175 pounds.) But our life together wasn't all calorie counting and exercising. We came up with planned indulgence days, when we would eat a little more or enjoy richer foods than usual. Because we scheduled those days in advance—and only occasionally—our eating never got out of control.

Today, I weigh 125 pounds—a weight I can maintain without starving myself or working out constantly. I look and feel better than ever. My back and joint pain and digestive problems are gone, and I breathe freely. Best of all, I have tons of energy and a positive attitude.

If I set my mind to something, I can do it.

Chapter 22

The Art of Emotional Self-Defense

Learning how to laugh at life's little irritations can save your health

All our lives, it seems, we dread the big disasters. Infidelity, a major illness, divorce. In comparison, life's minor irritations—the rude sales clerk, the driver who cuts us off on the highway, the wet towel a spouse leaves on the bathroom floor—seem like, well, minor irritations. Think again.

It's not just the big battles that kill. Studies have found that if you're constantly bent out of shape over petty, everyday problems, you may be as much as five times more likely to develop heart disease than those who are more laid back. You're also more likely to develop cancer and have high cholesterol and high blood pressure; and you're as much as seven times more likely to die prematurely from any cause.

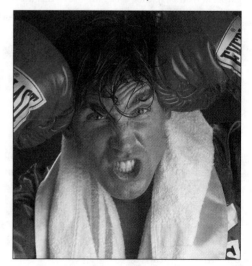

The Price We Pay

In some cases, scientists say, the relationship between getting mad at someone and harming your health is subtle: If you're feeling hostile or angry on a regular basis, you may drink more, smoke more, eat more, and exercise less. In other cases, it's more direct. Your emotions trigger a surge of stress hormones that cause your heart to pound faster, your blood to clot quicker, and your immune system to shut down. This leaves

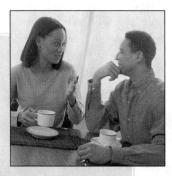

We Can Work It Out

Want to defuse conflicts you're having in a relationship? Practice the following communication techniques, suggest Redford Williams, M.D., director of behavioral-medicine research at Duke University Medical Center in Durham, North Carolina, and co-author of *Lifeskills* with Virginia Williams, Ph.D., who specializes in cultural history and social issues.

Open your mouth. Don't wait for the other person to initiate a discussion; speak up. Be specific and use simple sentences that start with "I" to tell the other person how you feel.

Use body language. Let your body show what you're feeling and thinking. Fifty percent of any message someone receives is nonverbal. So make sure your body and words are telling the same story. For example, crossing your arms defensively in front of your chest while you're telling someone why you're angry says that you're not ready to resolve anything.

Listen. Communication involves listening as well. During your exchange, figure that the other person is going to say things that may or may not make sense to you. "But listen to them," urges Dr. Redford Williams. "And keep in mind that you're not really listening unless you're prepared to be changed."

Practice assertion. State the problem: Describe your feelings and what you want. Describe the specific behavior that has caused your anger or hostility. Then request a specific change in the behavior that has upset you.

Empathize. Even if you think you're right, let the other person know that you appreciate his or her point of view. Then complete the sentence by repeating your request for a specific change in behavior.

you wide open for heart disease, cancer, and a host of chronic illnesses.

Are you helpless in the face of this self-inflicted emotional onslaught? Of course not.

Two doctors have developed a program called Lifeskills. It consists of simple, specific steps that can help you defeat the pernicious effects of life's little irritations.

Method for the Madness

Redford Williams is an M.D. who directs behavioral-medicine research at Duke University Medical Center in Durham, North Carolina. He also happens to be a pioneer in studying the effects of anger on health. Virginia Williams is a Ph.D. who specializes in cultural history and social issues. When they began experiencing tensions in their own 34-year marriage, they were in a better position than most to do something about it.

Here are the steps of the program they devised.

Identify your thoughts and feelings. Sounds simple, but there are so many layers and nuances to what you think and feel that sorting them out is hard. To make it easier, keep a pocket-size notebook at hand. Then, whenever you experience a less than loving moment with someone you care about, take a minute to write about the experience. Jot down five things.

> **NATURAL**FACT
>
> Body language counts. Fifty percent of the message we receive in a conversation is nonverbal.

1. A factual description of the encounter that has just taken place

2. What you thought during the encounter

3. What you felt

4. The actions you took

5. The consequences of those actions

Evaluate negative thoughts and feelings and your options. Now, carefully look at your notebook entry and ask yourself these questions.

• Is the matter important to me? Sometimes things really aren't worth getting upset about.

• Is what I'm thinking and feeling appropriate? What would you think if a friend came to you and related the same story?

• Is the situation modifiable? Is there anything you can do to change what happened?

• Is taking action worth it? When you balance your needs with those of others, will whatever you do improve or hurt your relationship?

Sometimes, just asking these questions can become a healthy way to counteract your negative feelings. It gives the part of your brain that may otherwise explode in anger something to wrestle with until its rational side catches up.

If you answered no to any of the questions, work on defusing your anger.

Solve the problem. Once you've identified the problem, brainstorm some solutions. Enlist friends in a brainstorming session to help find ways to cope with troubling situations or relationships.

Practice acceptance. When there's truly nothing you can do to turn around a relationship, another alternative is to simply accept the other person for who he or she is.

Communicate better. Unless you're a mind reader, you won't find out what another person is thinking or feeling unless they tell you. Similarly, you have to be willing to share what's on your mind.

Emphasize the positive. It's particularly important to have positive encounters while you're working on a specific problem, says Dr. Redford Williams. You may be dealing with some tough issues, and you don't want to feel like enemies.

Though it's likely true of most intimate relationships, studies of married couples show that it takes five positive encounters a day to cancel out the effects of one negative one, he says. In fact, that five-to-one ratio is so accurate that it can literally predict which marriages will succeed and which will slide toward divorce.

That's not to say that your relationship is on the skids if you talk about "troublesome truths" once in a while, he adds. But it is why you should frequently take time to smile, offer a hug, nuzzle a neck, or just share some milk and cookies.

NATURAL HEALING THROUGH HISTORY

Hildegard of Bingen: A Healer Ahead of Her Time

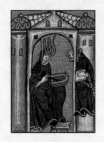

A saint, an herbalist, a medical genius, a visionary, a brilliant composer of spiritual music, a sex therapist, a scholar, and a leader of the church who corresponded with emperors, queens, and popes. All these achievements for any one person would be formidable. For a woman who lived virtually her entire life as a cloistered nun in the twelfth century, they are almost beyond belief.

Hildegard of Bingen was born of a noble German family in 1098. At the age of eight, she was committed to a monastery. Tutored by a neighboring monk in both classical and contemporary medical texts (at a time when most women couldn't read), she subsequently produced two major medical treatises of her own. One described the uses of more than 300 medicinal plants; another was a catalogue of diseases, their causes, and their cures.

Hildegard's healing philosophy was decidedly holistic. She wrote that the structure of the body echoed in miniature the sacred structure of the universe and that health resulted from being in harmony with that universal order. Her term for health was *greenness*, which she also described as "the green lifeforce of the flesh." She described the circulation of the blood, preached the virtues of a balanced, low-fat diet, and understood that disease was contagious—all hundreds of years ahead of her time.

Hildegard was also hundreds of years before her time in appreciating the connection between emotions and health. She understood that anger, for example, could give rise to "bile," which in turn could lead to disease. Recovery from illness required living a life that was in harmony, both with the natural world and with God's will. Sexuality was very much a part of that natural and divine order, Hildegard believed, and as a result, she described lovemaking in pious yet explicit terms. A man's passion, she wrote, is like "a stag thirsting for the fountain," while the woman resembles "a threshing floor, pounded by his many strokes and brought to heat when the grains are threshed inside her."

Since Hildegard was sworn to a vow of celibacy, it's assumed that her knowledge of such matters was based upon intimate conversations that she shared with married women from the communities surrounding her monastery.

Chapter 23

Shine a Light on the Bogeyman

How fear works—and how you can chase it from your life forever

Fear talks to us. It tells us we're crazy for getting on an airplane, for hiking in woods where bears might be hiding, for putting our hat in the ring for that big promotion. We all have that inner voice that whispers, and sometimes shouts, "Stop! You don't dare!"

The question is: How do you make that voice shut up?

Sometimes you don't want to. Fear isn't a character flaw—it's a survival mechanism. Without it, we'd be walking off cliffs and walking in front of cars. Often, though, fear only serves to hold us back, keeping us from doing the things we want to do—and *can* do.

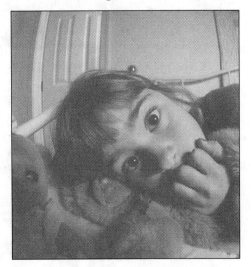

Don't let that happen. Learn fear's secrets, and use that knowledge to banish needless fear from your life.

Secret #1

It Doesn't Matter Why You're Scared

Strategy: **Stop searching the past.** You don't need to know exactly how or when you developed your fear of swimming or heights or thunderstorms to put that fear to rest. So why spend time and effort trying to figure it out? You're better off working on ways to overcome the fear.

"The stories we tell about how we've become fearful are often not true," says Steven E. Hyman, M.D., director of the National Institute of Mental Health (NIMH) in Bethesda, Maryland. "We just don't remember these things accurately, and they're not particularly helpful."

Secret #2

Fear Is Erased by Knowledge

Strategy: **Find out about what scares you.** If you know that the clunking sound that an airplane makes as it descends is the landing gear locking into position, rather than the wing falling off, you're less likely to run down the aisle screaming, "We're all going to die!"

"One of the main components to fear is uncertainty, or perhaps, more accurately,

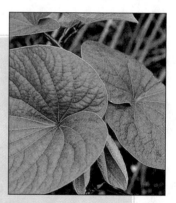

An Herb for Anxious Times

If modern life is leaving you stressed, anxiety-prone, or unable to sleep, kava kava may be the herb for you. "It allows relaxation while maintaining alertness," says Hyla Cass, M.D., assistant clinical professor of psychiatry at the University of California, Los Angeles, UCLA School of Medicine.

To use kava, Patricia Howell, a professional member of the American Herbalists Guild and director of the Living with Herbs Institute in Atlanta, advises starting out with ½ teaspoon of kava tincture (also called an extract) if you weigh between 130 and 175 pounds. Use a bit more or less if you fall under or over that range. "If you like the way the kava makes you feel, you can take another dose as soon as you feel the anxiety return," says Howell. Put the tincture in a little water and sip.

unpredictability," says S. J. Rachman, Ph.D., author of *Fear and Courage* and professor of psychology at the University of British Columbia in Vancouver. "When the situation becomes predictable, the fear diminishes."

This makes perfect sense when you realize that fear is a protective mechanism. In the absence of any other information, fear clicks on to steer you clear of a worst-case scenario. The more accurate and realistic your information is, the better this approach will work.

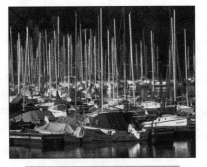

> **"Boats are safe in the harbor, but that's not what boats are made for."**
>
> —Anonymous

true. "People can pick up or model courageous or fearless behavior," says Dr. Rachman. "Watching somebody else behave bravely in a situation that's worrying you will definitely help." So if you're nervous about flying, plan a vacation with a friend who can be your courageous role model. Before your skiing lessons, spend some time watching the expert slopes.

Secret #3
Training Breeds Confidence

Strategy: **Be prepared.** It sounds simple, but it works. Rehearsal and practice help defuse anxiety. The army knows this, as do classical musicians, mountain climbers, and public speakers. "The closer the preparation comes to the actual situation, the more effective it is," Dr. Rachman says.

Secret #4
Courage Is Contagious

Strategy: **Catch it.** As anyone who has told ghost stories around a campfire knows, one jumpy person can give a whole group the jitters. But you may not realize that the opposite is also

Secret #5
Talking Helps

Strategy: **Open up.** It's hard to imagine anything more frightening than a terminal illness. "When you're looking at death, at its door, what I always suggest is to talk," says Alyssa Byrd, R.N., who counsels terminally ill patients at Lehigh Valley Hospice in Allentown, Pennsylvania. Similarly, when you're facing a major crisis, opening up about your fear can ease your distress even if you can't change the situation.

Conversely, trying to keep your fear under wraps isn't likely to help. "Suppressing fear is not a very effective technique," says Dr. Rachman.

Secret #6
Mind Games Work

Strategy: **Use your imagination.** Have a meeting coming up with someone who intimidates you? Bring him down to size by imagining him in his underwear. "This is a cognitive trick that changes the dominance ratio," says Richard Surwit, Ph.D., vice chair of research of the department of psychiatry and behavioral sciences at Duke University in Durham, North Carolina. When you're the only one dressed, you become the dominant one, and your fear goes away.

Secret #7
It's the Big Picture That's Scary

Strategy: Focus on the details. You've heard the saying about taking things "one day at a time"? That's what we're talking about here. "During intense fear, people tend to lose their focus on what they were doing and become overwhelmed," says Dr. Hyman. "The thing to do in this situation is to focus on the little things."

That means, get through your speech paragraph by paragraph; swim to shore stroke by stroke. Call it the don't-look-down principle: If you were walking a tightrope, you wouldn't look at the ground below you. You'd concentrate on putting one foot in front of the other until you got to the other side.

NATURALFACT

Some fears may have been with us so long that they've become almost instinctive. Fear of snakes, for example, turns up in people who've never seen a real one.

Secret #8
It's Okay to Get Help

Strategy: Seek counseling. When fear becomes an anxiety disorder, you may need to see a psychologist or psychiatrist to get over it. "If the feelings of fear are pervasive—you have them much of the day, most days, and they last for more than a few weeks—you should get treatment," Dr. Hyman says. One of the more severe anxiety disorders is panic disorder: panic attacks marked by sudden bouts of intense fear accompanied by rapid heartbeat and shortness of breath, often without an external cause.

But even if your fear isn't debilitating, you may find it useful to seek help if it's preventing you from doing what you want or need to do. "We're talking about 10 to 12 focused sessions aimed at getting rid of your symptoms," says Dr. Hyman. That's not to say that you can't beat your fears on your own, though. "As long as you don't have an out-of-control anxiety disorder, I think many people can face their fears and recognize that a lot of them are irrational." People can literally, by understanding what they're afraid of, make themselves braver.

Chapter 24

The Healing Power of Prayer

Science discovers miracles *do* happen; write your own spiritual prescription

After suffering from depression most of her life, Christine found herself, an atheist, asking for a sign from God. "I need to know I'm not alone," she prayed. "Is anybody there?"

At the time, she was sitting at the desk of her second floor office. Suddenly, something at the window caught her eye. It was a monarch butterfly, its black and orange wings glowing phosphorescently in the

morning sun. It fluttered at her window for a few minutes, then flew off.

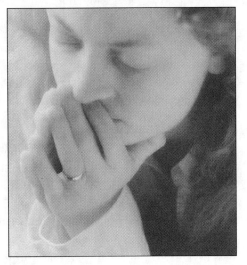

"I decided to take that as a yes," says Christine. "I didn't believe for a minute that it was a coincidence. In the 9 years I've been in that office, that was the first—and last—butterfly I ever saw at my window."

And it was also the last day that Christine suffered from depression.

"Wired for God"

What years of therapy and antidepressants couldn't cure, faith did.

Christine's sudden recovery once would have been scoffed at by doctors as just another manifestation of her neurosis. But today, they're more likely to take notice. That's because solid medical research has uncovered one of the greatest healing miracles of all time in what is both the most unlikely—and likely—of places: church.

Christine's cure would come as no surprise to Harold G. Koenig, M.D., director of the Duke University Center for the Study of Religion, Spirituality, and Health in Durham, North Carolina, and author of *The Healing Power of Faith*. In his study of 87 seriously depressed men and women conducted at Duke University Medical Center, he found that those who put spirituality at the center of their lives recovered 70 percent faster than those who didn't. And the more spiritually centered an individual was, the faster he or she healed.

A second study, involving 1,700 people over the age of 65, compared immune system factors in those who attended religious services with those who didn't. Dr. Koenig found that those who went to services—even just once a month—had significantly stronger immune systems.

Twenty years ago, Dr. Koenig couldn't pay scientific audiences to listen to him talk about connections between spirituality and health. But today, he's in such demand as a speaker that he shuttles from coast to coast with barely enough time to change his shirt. "For many years, scientists thought spirituality was something only neurotic people pursued," Dr. Koenig explains. "But now we're finding evidence that maybe spirituality is part of what it is to be human, and that it may work together with our individual psy-

The Scientific Evidence

The healing power of faith is supported by some impressive research from some impressive academic institutions. For example:

- A study at the California Public Health Foundation in Berkeley that followed more than 5,000 people for 28 years found that the risk of dying prematurely among women who went to church once a week or more was one-third less than that of women who did not. And that's after taking into account smoking, drinking, exercise, and weight, which are all factors related to physical health.

- Cardiac surgery patients who said they received "strength and comfort" from their faith were three times more likely to survive than those who did not, according to a study of 232 men and women done at the Dartmouth-Hitchcock

chology to indirectly affect our health."

In fact, Herbert Benson, M.D., associate professor of medicine at Harvard Medical School and president of the Mind/Body Medical Institute at New England Deaconess Hospital in Boston, suggests that because faith plays such an influential role in health, it makes sense that humans must be "wired for God": genetically programmed to believe, if not in a being called God, at least in a power greater than ourselves. In his work identifying the

Medical Center in Lebanon, New Hampshire.

- In a study of 112 women, researchers at the University of North Carolina in Greensboro reported a link between high "religiosity" and lower blood pressure, even when lifestyle factors such as weight, smoking, alcohol use, and diet were taken into account. In fact, being religious had an even stronger beneficial effect on the women's blood pressures than other health habits, good or bad.

- A landmark study of nearly 92,000 Maryland residents by researchers at Johns Hopkins University in Baltimore found that weekly churchgoers died 50 percent less often from heart disease, emphysema, and suicide, and 74 percent less often from cirrhosis than people who did not attend church as often.

- Of 393 men and women admitted to the cardiac care unit at San

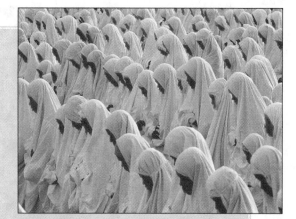

Francisco General Hospital, those who were prayed for—even though they had no idea that anyone was praying for them—were five times less likely to require antibiotics and six times less likely to need artificial ventilation treatment.

- A 16-year study of 11 religious and 11 secular kibbutzim (Israeli communal settlements) by researchers at Hadassah University and Ben-Gurion University in Israel revealed that religious Jews of all ages were half as likely to die from any cause during the study as Jews who did not practice their faith.

stress-reducing "relaxation response," he discovered that people who meditate are healthy, but those who experience spirituality as a result are healthier.

Why Faith Helps

The evidence that spirituality heals is impressive. More than 300 studies have found that people of faith are healthier than nonbelievers and less likely to die prematurely from any cause. Having faith can also speed recovery from physical and mental illness, surgery, and addiction.

There are a host of reasons why, says Dale A. Matthews, M.D., associate professor of medicine at Georgetown University School of Medicine in Washington, D.C., and author of *The Faith Factor: Proof of the Healing Power of Prayer.* Among them are the following items.

• The body responds positively to faith. People who regularly practice their religious beliefs have healthier results on tests of their blood pressures, breathing, pulses, and immune systems than people who don't, Dr. Matthews says.

• Faith produces a peaceful state of mind and hopefulness. Such an outlook can reduce stress, anxiety, and depression.

• Religious people tend to take better care of themselves. They are less likely to drink and smoke, and they're more likely to take their medicines and wear seat belts than nonreligious people, notes Dr. Matthews.

• Being enmeshed in a faith community is healthy. Numerous studies have shown the healing power of social ties. For many people, the church, temple, or mosque is "family," the place where they feel a sense of connection, meaning, and purpose, says Dr. Matthews. "They're surrounded by people who share the same beliefs they do, people who call them when they don't attend worship, visit them when they're in the hospital, and even bake them cookies and casseroles when they return home."

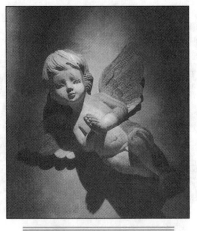

> "For many years, scientists thought spirituality was something only neurotic people pursued. Now we're finding evidence that maybe spirituality is part of what it is to be human."
>
> —Harold G. Koenig, M.D.

An Ecumenical Effect

Obviously, church isn't the only route to physical well-being. People with no religious beliefs what-soever can stay healthy by meditating, exercising, having a positive attitude, taking care of themselves, and having friends. Dr. Matthews maintains, however, that religion is more powerful because it combines the basics of a healthy lifestyle with something greater: faith in the helping hand of God.

Most of the studies on the healing power of faith thus far have examined Christians, but that doesn't mean Christians are the only ones who can enjoy the fruits of spiritual belief. "It's likely that the effects also apply to Muslims, Jews, and others of monotheistic faiths," says Dr. Koenig. "The only reason I wouldn't say it applies to still other religions is that we just don't have enough data yet."

But Dr. Benson, who feels he has seen enough data, says firmly, "It does not matter which God you worship, nor which theology you adopt. Spiritual life, in general, is very healthy."

Ruth Baker is living, healthy proof. A 51-year-old teacher, Ruth has suffered from a chronic pain condition for much of her life. In fact, says Ruth, she would still suffer from it if she did not practice zazen, a Buddhist meditation in which she contemplates the meaning of a koan (word puzzle) for an hour every day.

"I sit down in a room by myself for 45 minutes every morning and work on the koan," she says. "I repeat it silently to myself as I slowly breathe in, then exhale. It interrupts my ordinary interior dialogue, so that I stop habitual patterns of thinking and become one with the moment. Afterward, I walk around the room for another 15 minutes, still contemplating the koan. By the time I'm finished, my emotional pitch has dropped. I become much quieter inside, which allows me to become more relaxed and accepting of my pain. And that allows the pain to diminish."

Cultivating Your Connection

You can't suddenly "have faith" simply to prolong your life or help you recover from an illness. Being religious or spiritual isn't a good health habit such as eating more vegetables, lacing up your running shoes, or even meditating. Research shows that one of the key ingredients is that your desire to develop spiritually "comes from the heart," says Dave Larson, M.D., a former National Institutes of Health researcher who now heads the privately funded National Institute for Healthcare Research.

Just going through the motions doesn't do it, agrees Dr. Koenig. The guy who goes to church to network and make business contacts or the woman who joins a neighborhood prayer circle just to meet the right people probably won't achieve health and longevity through the experience. There's even some evidence to show that using religion in this way is actually associated with worse mental health.

But if you're drawn to spirituality, or would like to further develop your own faith, here are a few suggestions for making it a part of your life.

Give faith a chance. If you're only in your place of worship for weddings and funerals or if your previous religious experience wasn't satisfying, you may wonder how to get spirituality into your life. Keep an open mind, says Dr. Koenig. "I'm not suggesting that people go to church or turn to religion. I'm just suggesting that you be open to the notion of religion and spirituality. Ask yourself, 'Have I really given spirituality a chance?' Even if you've dismissed it before, be open to the role that spirituality or God might play in your life." Your quest is likely to draw you to a religion or spir-

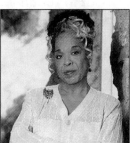

HEALING SPOTLIGHT
Della Reese

Della Reese plays the loving angel Tess on TV's *Touched by an Angel*, but for her, faith is far more than an act. Twice she was saved by God from life-threatening illness, she says: once when she was seriously injured in an accident and once when a blood vessel ruptured in her brain. Those experiences and others taught her never to doubt what God can do.

"I have advice for people going through hard times, good times, or whatever times," Reese says. "God is good all the time, so trust him."

itual community where you do feel comfortable.

Say a little prayer. "The easiest way to begin is often with a centering prayer or the relaxation response form of prayer," says Dr. Matthews. See "A Peaceful Prayer" for a description of how to pray meditatively.

Read the good word. Pick a reading from your own religious tradition or one that appeals to you and read it every day for 15 to 20 minutes, suggests Dr. Matthews. "I've found early morning is best because it allows me to prepare for the day by grounding myself in God and finding sustenance to help buffer life's stresses."

Join a spiritual community. "Attend worship services on a regular basis and get involved with small groups within a spiritual community," says Dr. Matthews. Join the community's women's or men's group, choir, urban outreach mission, or soup kitchen. Continual involvement is likely to mean continual benefit.

Get in touch with your religious roots. Most religions have their own healing

NATURALFACT

More than one-third of the nation's medical schools now offer courses on spirituality and health as either requirements or electives.

traditions—ceremonies, prayers, and rituals that offer comfort and hope to the sick and distressed. Recovering some of these past traditions can bring you untold benefits, as Rabbi Simkha Weintraub, rabbinic director of the National Center for Jewish Healing in New York City, can attest. "Jews today are just beginning to recover the old prayers, meditations, and rituals that didn't originally come to light as part of the bare-bones Judaism that survived major disruptions such as the Holocaust."

A tradition that Rabbi Weintraub finds healing is one in which a spiritual community organizes a group of people—a *Hevrah*—to recite the book of Psalms (*Tehillim*) when someone is seriously ill. For example, when another rabbi's wife had breast cancer not too long ago, his congregation organized a Hevrah Tehillim every day while she was being treated. They also prepared meals for the family, carpooled the kids, and generally helped out. "The congregation deepened itself in a profound way," says Rabbi Weintraub. "And the Hevrah Tehillim provided great support for everyone."

A Peaceful Prayer

Never tried "centering prayer"? Relax—it's easy. And relaxing.

Sit in a quiet room, close your eyes, and take a deep breath, imagining that the breath is coming from your toes. Then, as you exhale, focus your mind on a word that symbolizes your spirituality: "God," "Allah," "shalom," or "Jesus" are examples. Your mind will tend to wander, but that's okay. Just gently bring it back to your chosen word.

Repeat the word silently to yourself with each exhalation for the next 15 to 20 minutes. Then slowly open your eyes. Try to do this once or twice every day.

NATURAL HEALING IN THE FUTURE

Heart to Heart

Dean Ornish, M.D., became famous as the heart doctor who proved that a low-fat diet, daily exercise, and stress-reduction techniques could reverse heart disease. Now he's taking his no-drugs, no-surgery philosophy to the next level. Here, Dr. Ornish describes the holistic view of health 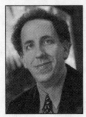 that will dominate the next century.

Q: You've written a book called *Love and Survival: The Scientific Basis for the Healing Power of Intimacy*. Could you explain what kind of love you're talking about? You don't just mean romantic love, right?

A: Right. Love can be a manifestation of romantic intimacy. But it can also be a manifestation of intimacy between you and your family, you and your friends, or you and members of your community. It can be between you and a pet. It can reflect intimacy between you and parts of yourself that you're not in touch with. It can even be a spiritual experience.

The idea is that although we're all separate individuals, we're also part of something larger that connects us all. And anything that takes you out of the experience of being separate is healing.

Q: You say in your book that these feelings of isolation and depression are virtu-

ally epidemic in today's society. Why do you think that's true?

A: There's been a radical shift in our culture in the last 50 years. We've seen a breakdown of the family. Many people don't have a job, church, synagogue, or neighborhood that they've been a part of for very long.

Awareness is the first step in healing. I wrote this book to show what a difference love and intimacy can make, not only in the quality of our lives but also in our survival, so that we can make different choices. Spending time with friends and loved ones is a basic human need, as basic as eating, breathing, and sleeping. That need so often goes unfulfilled in our culture. And that threatens our survival.

Q: You talk a lot in your book about the importance of relationships, support groups, and therapy, but you also describe meditation and prayer as paths to healing and joy. Aren't those solitary, isolating activities?

A: Prayer and meditation can give you the direct experience of transcendence and a higher level of interconnectedness with others. I define love and intimacy as anything that takes you out of the experience of being separate. And a powerful way to do that is to commune with God, or whatever name you give to that experience.

Herbs and Essential Oils

While herbal home remedies are generally safe and cause few, if any, side effects, herbalists are quick to note that botanical medicines should be used cautiously and knowledgeably. If you are under a doctor's care for any health condition or are taking any medication, don't take any herb or use any essential oils without your doctor knowing about it. Some herbs and oils may cause adverse reactions if you are allergy-prone, have a major health condition, take prescription medication, take an herb or use an oil for too long, take too much, or use the herb or oil improperly. If you are pregnant, nursing, or trying to conceive, do not self-treat yourself with any natural remedy without the consent of your obstetrician or midwife.

Essential oils are inhaled or placed on the skin but never taken internally because they are so concentrated that they can be toxic. Never apply essential oils undiluted unless otherwise indicated. Dilute them first in a neutral base, which can be an oil (such as almond), cream, or gel before application. Many essential oils may cause skin irritation or allergic reaction in people with sensitive skin. Before applying any new oil to your skin, always do a patch test. Put a few drops of diluted oil on the back of your wrist. Wait for an hour or more. If irritation or redness occur, bathe the area with cold water. For future use, prepare a dilution with half the amount of essential oil or avoid it altogether. Store essential oils in dark bottles, away from light or heat, and out of the reach of children and pets.

Check these safety guidelines, which are based on the advice of experienced herbal healers, before you try the remedies in this book. Below are cautions for the herbs and essential oils mentioned in this book that can potentially cause adverse reactions in some people. Though such occurrences are rare, you should be aware of what they are and discontinue the use of the herb if you experience an unusual reaction. Also, do not exceed the recommended dosage—more is not better. With this in mind, you can enjoy the world of herbal healing with confidence.

Herb (Botanical Name)	Safety Guidelines
ALOE (*ALOE BARBADENSIS*)	May delay wound healing; do not use gel externally on any surgical incision; do not ingest the dried leaf, as it is a habit-forming laxative
ANGELICA (*ANGELICA ARCHANGELICA*)	Use sparingly and only for short periods of time; increases sun sensitivity
ARNICA (*ARNICA MONTANA*)	Do not use on broken skin
ASHWAGANDA (*WITHANIA SOMNIFERA*)	Do not use with barbiturates because it may intensify their effects
BASIL (*OCIMUM BASILICUM*)	Do not take large amounts (several cups a day) for extended periods

Herb (Botanical Name)	Safety Guidelines
BIRCH (*BETULA* SPP.)	Do not take if you need to avoid aspirin because its active ingredient, salicin, is related to aspirin
BLACK COHOSH (*CIMICIFUGA RACEMOSA*)	Do not use for more than 6 months
BLACK HAW (*VIBURNUM PRUNIFOLIUM*)	Do not take without medical supervision if you have a history of kidney stones as it contains oxalates, which can cause kidney stones
BORAGE (*BORAGO OFFICINALIS*)	For external use only; long-term use is not recommended
BROMELAIN	Bromelain may cause nausea, vomiting, diarrhea, skin rash, and heavy menstrual bleeding; do not use it if you are allergic to pineapple; bromelain could increase the risk of bleeding in patients taking aspirin or other blood-thinning drugs
CASCARA SAGRADA (*RHAMNUS PURSHIANUS*)	Do not use if you have any inflammatory condition of the intestines, intestinal obstruction, or abdominal pain; can cause laxative dependency and diarrhea; don't use for more than 14 days
CHAMOMILE (*MATRICARIA RECUTITA*)	Very rarely, can cause an allergic reaction when ingested; people allergic to closely related plants such as ragweed, asters, and chrysanthemums should drink the tea with caution
CHASTEBERRY (*VITEX AGNUS-CASTUS*)	May counteract the effectiveness of birth control pills
COMFREY (*SYMPHYTUM OFFICINALE*)	For external use only; do not use topically on deep or infected wounds because it can promote surface healing too quickly and not allow healing of underlying tissue
DANDELION (*TARAXACUM OFFICINALE*)	If you have gallbladder disease, do not use dandelion root preparations without medical approval
ECHINACEA (*ECHINACEA ANGUSTIFOLIA, E. PURPUREA, E. PALLIDA*)	Do not use if allergic to closely related plants such as ragweed, asters, and chrysanthemums; do not use if you have tuberculosis or an autoimmune condition such as lupus or multiple sclerosis because echinacea stimulates the immune system
EPHEDRA (*EPHEDRA SINICA*)	Use only with a qualified health practitioner
EUCALYPTUS (*EUCALYPTUS GLOBULUS*)	Do not use if you have inflammatory disease of the bile ducts or gastrointestinal tract or severe liver disease; may cause nausea, vomiting, and diarrhea in doses higher than 4 grams a day
FENNEL (*FOENICULUM VULGARE*)	Do not use medicinally for more than 6 weeks without supervision by a qualified herbalist
FEVERFEW (*CHRYSANTHEMUM PARTHENIUM; TANACETUM PARTHENIUM*)	Fresh leaves can cause mouth sores in some people if chewed
FLAX (*LINUM USITATISSIMUM*)	Do not take if you have a bowel obstruction; take with at least 8 ounces of water
GARLIC (*ALLIUM SATIVUM*)	Do not use supplements if you're on anticoagulants or before undergoing surgery because garlic thins the blood and may increase bleeding; do not use if you're taking hypoglycemic drugs

Herb (Botanical Name)	Safety Guidelines
GENTIAN (*GENTIANA LUTEA*)	May cause nausea and vomiting in large doses; do not use if you have high blood pressure, gastric or duodenal ulcers, or gastric irritation and inflammation
GINGER (*ZINGIBER OFFICINALE*)	May increase bile secretion, so if you have gallstones, do not use therapeutic amounts of the dried root or powder without guidance from a health-care practitioner
GINKGO (*GINKGO BILOBA*)	Do not use with antidepressant MAO inhibitor drugs such as phenelzine sulfate (Nardil) or tranylcypromine (Parnate), aspirin or other nonsteroidal anti-inflammatory medications, or blood-thinning medications such as warfarin (Coumadin); can cause dermatitis, diarrhea, and vomiting in doses higher than 240 milligrams of concentrated extract
GOLDENSEAL (*HYDRASTIS CANADENSIS*)	Do not use if you have high blood pressure
GUGGUL (*COMMIPHORA MUKUL*)	Rarely, may trigger diarrhea, restlessness, apprehension, or hiccups
HAWTHORN (*CRATAEGUS OXYCANTHA*; *C. LAEVIGATA*; *C. MONOGYNA*)	If you have a cardiovascular condition, do not take hawthorn regularly for more than a few weeks without medical supervision. You may require lower doses of other medications, such as high blood pressure drugs; if you have low blood pressure caused by heart valve problems, do not use without medical supervision
HOPS (*HUMULUS LUPULUS*)	Do not take if prone to depression; rarely, can cause skin rash, so handle fresh or dried hops carefully
HORSE CHESTNUT (*AESCULUS HIPPOCASTANUM*)	May interfere with the action of other drugs, especially blood thinners such as warfarin (Coumadin); may irritate the gastrointestinal tract
HORSETAIL (*EQUISETUM* SPP.)	Do not use tincture if you have heart or kidney problems; may cause a thiamin deficiency; do not take more than 2 grams per day of powdered extract or take for prolonged periods
KAVA KAVA (*PIPER METHYSTICUM*)	Do not take with alcohol or barbiturates; do not take more than the recommended dose on package; use caution when driving or operating equipment as this herb is a muscle relaxant
KOREAN GINSENG; OFTEN REFERRED TO AS GINSENG (*PANAX GINSENG*)	May cause irritability if taken with caffeine or other stimulants; do not take if you have high blood pressure
LICORICE (*GLYCYRRHIZA GLABRA*)	Do not use if you have diabetes, high blood pressure, liver or kidney disorders, or low potassium levels; do not use daily for more than 4 to 6 weeks because overuse can lead to water retention, high blood pressure caused by potassium loss, or impaired heart and kidney function
MARSHMALLOW (*ALTHAEA OFFICINALIS*)	May slow the absorption of medications taken at the same time
NETTLE (*URTICA DIOICA*)	If you have allergies, your symptoms may worsen, so take only one dose a day for the first few days
OATSTRAW; ALSO OATS (*AVENA SATIVA*)	Do not use if you have celiac disease (gluten intolerance), as it contains gluten, a grain protein

Herb (Botanical Name)	Safety Guidelines
PARSLEY (*PETROSELINUM CRISPUM*)	If you have kidney disease, do not use large amounts (several cups a day) because it increases urine flow; safe as a garnish or ingredient in food
PYGEUM (*PYGEUM AFRICANUM*)	May cause nausea and stomach pain
ROSEMARY (*ROSMARINUS OFFICINALIS*)	May cause excessive menstrual bleeding
SAGE (*SALVIA OFFICINALIS*)	Used in therapeutic amounts, can increase sedative side effects of drugs; do not use if you're hypoglycemic or undergoing anticonvulsant therapy
ST. JOHN'S WORT (*HYPERICUM PERFORATUM*)	Do not use with antidepressants without medical approval; may cause photosensitivity; avoid overexposure to direct sunlight
SASSAFRAS (*SASSAFRAS ALBIDUM*)	Long-term use is not recommended; do not take more than the recommended dose
SAW PALMETTO (*SERENOA REPENS*)	Consult your doctor if using to treat an enlarged prostate
SENNA (*CASSIA SENNA*)	Do not use if you have a bowel obstruction; take 1 hour after other drugs; take with at least 8 ounces of water
TURMERIC (*CURCUMA DOMESTICA*)	Do not use as a home remedy if you have high stomach acid or ulcers, gallstones, or bile duct obstruction
VALERIAN (*VALERIANA OFFICINALIS*)	Do not use with sleep-enhancing or mood-regulating medications because it may intensify their effects; may cause heart palpitations and nervousness in sensitive individuals; if such stimulant action occurs, discontinue use
WHITE WILLOW (*SALIX ALBA*)	Do not take if you need to avoid aspirin, especially if you are taking blood-thinning medication such as warfarin (Coumadin) because its active ingredient is related to aspirin; may interact with barbiturates or sedatives such as aprobarbital (Amytal) or alprazolam (Xanax); can cause stomach irritation when consumed with alcohol; do not give to children under age 16 who have any viral infection; may contribute to Reye's syndrome, which affects the brain and liver
YARROW (*ACHILLEA MILLEFOLIUM*)	Rarely, handling flowers can cause skin rash
YELLOW DOCK (*RUMEX CRISPUS*)	If you have a history of kidney stones, do not take without medical supervision, as it contains oxalates and tannins that may adversely affect this condition
YOHIMBE (*PAUSINYSTALIA YOHIMBE*)	Use only with a qualified health practitioner

Essential Oils	Safety Guidelines
BAY	Use in moderation and not for more than 2 weeks without the guidance of a qualified practitioner
BERGAMOT	Avoid direct sunlight after topical application because skin sensitivity can occur (except bergapten-free type)
CINNAMON	Do not use for more than 2 weeks without the guidance of a qualified practitioner
CLOVE	Use in moderation and not for more than 2 weeks without the guidance of a qualified practitioner; can be used undiluted for tooth pain

Essential Oils	Safety Guidelines
EUCALYPTUS	Use in moderation and not for more than 2 weeks without the guidance of a qualified practitioner
LAUREL	Use in moderation and not for more than 2 weeks without the guidance of a qualified practitioner because it causes lethargy and unconsciousness
LAVENDER	Can be used undiluted, but keep it away from your eyes
LEMON	Avoid direct sunlight after topical application because skin sensitivity can occur
LEMONGRASS	Topical use only—don't inhale
RAVENSARA	Do not use for more than 2 weeks without the guidance of a qualified practitioner
ROSEMARY	Do not use if you have hypertension (high blood pressure); do not use if you have epilepsy, due to the powerful action on the nervous system
SAGE (CLARY)	Do not use with alcohol because it can cause a narcotic effect and exaggerate drunkenness
SANDALWOOD	Can be used undiluted as a perfume, but keep it away from your eyes
TEA TREE	May be applied undiluted to the skin

Credits

Cover photograph

© by Hilmar, 1999

Interior photographs

Courtesy of Mark Blumenthal: page 155

© Wayne H. Chasan/The Image Bank: page xvi

Rob Cardillo/Rodale Images: page 72

Chas Bush Stock: page 7

Corbis/Gianni Dagli Orti: page 150

Corbis/Araldo de Luca: page 168

Corbis/ Werner Forman: page 39

Corbis/Mimmo Jodice: page 13

Corbis/Tom Nebbia: page 199

Corbis/Roger Ressmeyer: page 61

© by Gabriel M. Covan/The Image Bank: page 66

Tim DeFrisco/Rodale Images: page 182

© by Tom Devol: page 203

Robert Gerheart/Rodale Images: page 59

Tom Gettings/Rodale Images: page 152

© by Greg Gorman: page 32

Gilbert S. Grant/PhotoResearchers: page 212

Michael Grecco/SYGMA: page 163

John P. Hamel/Rodale Images: pages xv, 8, 17, 22, 63, 79, 90, 100, 109, 121, 125, 132, 148, 198, 206, and 213

Courtesy of The Honorable Tom Harkin, The Senate of the United States: page 56

Courtesy of Clare Hastler: page 99

© by Hilmar: pages 28, 29, 40, 180, and 195

Ed Landrock/Rodale Images: pages 4, 75, 78, 82, 112, and 178

© by Catherine Ledner: page 102

Erich Lessing/Art Resource, NY: page 210

© by Cliff Lipson/CBS: page 219

Mitch Mandel/Rodale Images: pages 14, 15, 18, 30, 43, 48, 62, 67, 87, 90, 117, 156, 161, 169, 170, 196, and 211

John McDonough/Sports Illustrated, © by Time Inc.: page 201

PhotoDisc: pages 17, 77, 215, 217, and 218

© by H. Lee Puckett: page 110

© by Bill Reitzel: page 221

Rodale Images: pages 2, 12, 19, 23, 57, 70, 83, 97, 104, 114, 119, 123, 139, 142, 143, 145, 151, 153, 162, 176, 187, 188, 196, 198, 206, 207, 211, 212, and 213

© by John Sterling Ruth: page 25

Margret Skrovanek/Rodale Images: page 137

Courtesy of Judith Stern: page 69

Tony Stone Images/Hutton Getty: page 186

Susan Vogel: page 45

Tad Ware & Company: page 81

Courtesy of Lynne Watson: page 204

Kurt Wilson/Rodale Images: pages 9, 21, 26, 34, 37, 41, 46, 49, 51, 52, 73, 78, 84, 93, 95, 103, 106, 119, 127, 158, 159, 164, 166, 172, and 207

Courtesy of Susan Yanovski: page 175

Illustrations

Scott Angle: pages 190–194

INDEX

Underscored references indicate boxed text.